W9-APF-139

Women'sHealth

The 12-Week
Head-to-Toe
Transformation

Women'sHealth

The 12-Week
Head-to-Toe
Transformation

A Beginner's Guide to
Fitness & Strength Training
in **3** Simple Steps

Holly Perkins, CSCS

RODALE

This book is intended as a reference volume only, not as a medical manual. The information given here is designed to help you make informed decisions about your health. It is not intended as a substitute for any treatment that may have been prescribed by your doctor. If you suspect that you have a medical problem, we urge you to seek competent medical help.

The information in this book is meant to supplement, not replace, proper exercise training. All forms of exercise pose some inherent risks. The editors and publisher advise readers to take full responsibility for their safety and know their limits. Before practicing the exercises in this book, be sure that your equipment is well-maintained, and do not take risks beyond your level of experience, aptitude, training, and fitness. The exercise and dietary programs in this book are not intended as a substitute for any exercise routine or dietary regimen that may have been prescribed by your doctor. As with all exercise and dietary programs, you should get your doctor's approval before beginning.

Mention of specific companies, organizations, or authorities in this book does not imply endorsement by the author or publisher, nor does mention of specific companies, organizations, or authorities imply that they endorse this book, its author, or the publisher.

Internet addresses and telephone numbers given in this book were accurate at the time it went to press.

The direct online and trade editions were published simultaneously in April 2015 as *Women's Health Lift to Get Lean*.

© 2015 by Rodale Inc.
Photographs © 2015 by Rodale Inc.

All rights reserved. No part of this publication may be reproduced or transmitted in any form or by any means, electronic or mechanical, including photocopying, recording, or any other information storage and retrieval system, without the written permission of the publisher.

Rodale books may be purchased for business or promotional use or for special sales. For information, please write to:
Special Markets Department, Rodale Inc., 733 Third Avenue, New York, NY 10017

Women's Health is a registered trademark of Rodale Inc.

Printed in China

Photographs by Tom MacDonald/Rodale Images
Book design by Joanna Williams

Library of Congress Cataloging-in-Publication Data is on file with the publisher.

ISBN 978-1-62336-478-6   trade paperback
ISBN 978-1-62336-479-3   direct online hardcover

Distributed to the trade by Macmillan

2 4 6 8 10 9 7 5 3   trade paperback

4 6 8 10 9 7 5   direct online hardcover

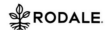

We inspire health, healing, happiness, and love in the world.
Starting with you.

To Trampas and Josey,
for loving me long before I truly knew
how to love myself

Contents

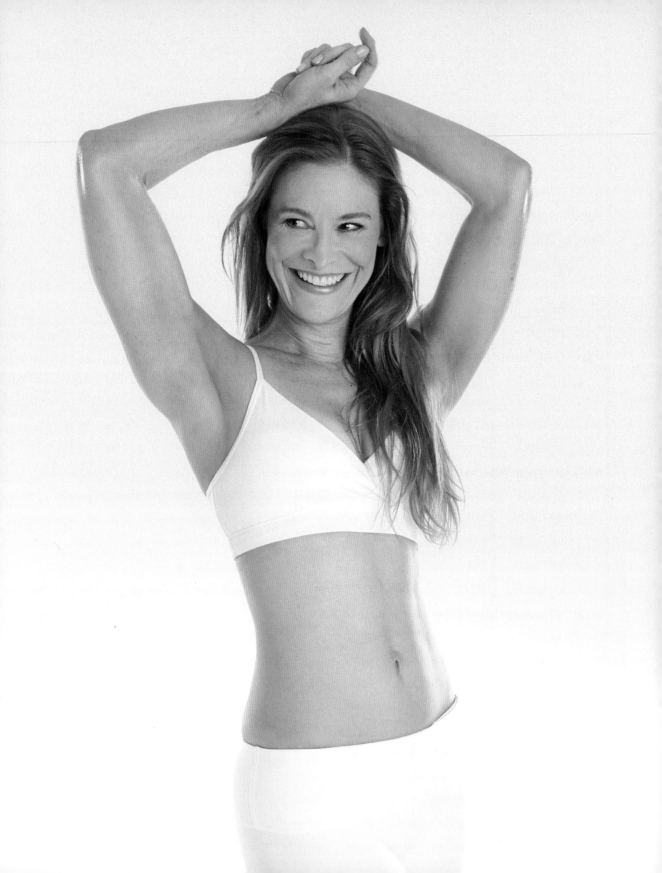

Introduction

Change Your Body, Change Your Life

Psst! Holly Perkins here and I have a confession to make right off the bat. It's about the cover of this book, *The 12-Week Head-to-Toe Transformation.* Well, you see, that's not my favorite title.

If I had my way, a far more accurate title would be *Women's Health Lift to Get Lean . . . and Strong . . . and Healthy . . . and Confident . . . and Happy . . . and Energetic . . . and Fearless . . . and Capable of Achieving Everything You Put Your Mind To.*

Unfortunately my editor nixed those—something about lack of cover space and how the word "transformation" is more compelling—but you get the idea. This book—which includes my complete Lift to Get Lean program— will change much more than your body. It will change your whole life.

I know it seems like a list of bold promises, but I believe in every one of them completely and wholeheartedly because I have experienced them myself, and I know you can, too. This book will give you the exact tools you need to develop the lean, toned body of your dreams. And it will help you tap into your personal strength.

This book is about *you* using the practice of strength training to become strong in every aspect of your life. Therefore, going forward, I have made a very intentional decision to refer to this practice as "strength training" rather than

"weight lifting" or even "resistance training." The strength that you will cultivate is physical, emotional, mental, and spiritual. Word choice may seem incon-
sequential to some, but I feel that the language we use on a regular basis has a
great impact on our lives. Start your morning saying, "I'm going to have a great
day today," and chances are it's going to turn out pretty good. So when you exercise, you will *strength* train. Use the words *strength* and *strong* and you'll make it
happen. I truly believe that.

For the past 20 years, I have been a sought-after personal trainer, working
daily with Hollywood's elite: actors, models, producers, business owners, professional athletes, executives, moms, and politicians. And all of my experience has
taught me one thing: In order to help you become *lean,* I need to help you become
strong. The path to becoming the lean, gorgeous, confident machine that you're
meant to be is through strength training.

So welcome to my sphere of strength! In my world, working out is a metaphor
for life. And the gym is a playground where you will discover your abilities,
achieve what you thought was impossible, and push through the weight of your
world. In this playground, you can define who you are, what you want, and how
you want to live.

Busting the Bulky Myth

Now, before we head off on this journey, I want to address a common female con-
cern about this particular playground. Despite the information age that we live
in, many women still harbor unfounded fears of "bulking up" from lifting
weights. They feel—and maybe you do, too—that exercising with barbells, dumbbells, and strength-training machines will make them muscle-bound and mas-
culine. At the same time, most women also have a deep desire to feel tight, lean,
and fit but have never experienced what it feels like to move through a normal
day in a body that is strong and resilient. It's an amazing feeling, and I want
you to experience it. But the only way to get there is to defeat this fear of the
"bulking-up boogieman" and start strength training in earnest.

Because of the misinformation in the fitness industry, many women have thrown up their hands in a gesture of "I give up." They have abandoned their goals of being fit and lean because they are confused and afraid. They have come to believe that their bodies don't respond to "toning" exercises because they haven't found a system that works.

Can you relate?

Research proves that it is physiologically impossible for women to bulk up (a process called hypertrophy) in the first 6 weeks of a strength-training program. As a woman, you simply do not have enough testosterone (the so-called male hormone) coursing through your body to pack on big muscle that quickly the way your boyfriend can. What's more, the way you will be training on my program will create beautiful muscle tone, not Incredible Hulk bulk (nor green skin)! And you will experience recognizable changes in your body in the first 6 weeks. This is the critical time in a program when many women get scared and abandon their goals of becoming strong. But *you* won't.

I have created a system that ensures you develop functional strength without adding muscle size unless you really want to. Every day I hear clients say that they actually feel good and enjoy their time spent in the gym for once in their lives. This book will inspire you to adopt a new approach to fitness; to think differently about strength training; and to quit worrying, once and for all, that you will bulk up from lifting weights.

The Biggest Problem in Women's Fitness Today

This book is an introduction to proper strength training for women. After many years of close examination, I realized that the biggest problem with the current landscape of women's fitness is that men have dictated the rules in the gym. Weight-lifting and gym workouts are the hallmark of athletes and sports teams in a male-dominated industry. Until now, women have looked to men for workouts, exercises, and general weight-lifting information.

There is a problem with this standard, though: Women's bodies are different from men's bodies.

> Because of hormonal differences, women respond differently to strength training.

> Because of structural differences, women will add muscle in different places than men.

> Women have very different functional and aesthetic preferences compared to men.

> Women have very different motivators.

These factors alone mean that a woman's body will respond in a unique way to her strength-training workouts. And, as you'll learn, the female body responds exceptionally well to strength training.

The Whole-Body Health Solution

I know without a doubt that strength training will change your body in profound ways. In fact, I will go so far as to say that strength training is as critical to your health as Pap tests, mammograms, and annual visits to your doctor. Strength training is one of the most powerful tools you can use to directly influence your overall health and general sense of well-being. I'll give you scientific proof about the benefits of strength training in Chapter 5, but here's a quick preview to whet your appetite. These are the rewards you can expect to gain by strength training the Lift to Get Lean way.

> Strength training will trim your body faster than any other exercise.

> Strength training will recharge your resting metabolism so you'll burn more calories, even while asleep, and it will help you maintain your weight loss.

> Strength training will protect you from osteoporosis (brittle bones) as you get older by boosting your bone mineral density.

> Strength training will reverse muscle loss that occurs each year after age 30. Why is retaining muscle important? See the second bullet above. Muscle is more metabolically active (i.e., calorie-burning) than fat is.

> Strength training will put a spring in your step and make you more energetic and athletic.

> Strength training will help you stick to healthy eating habits.

> Strength training will reduce your risk of developing insulin resistance and type 2 diabetes.

> Strength training may keep your heart muscle healthy and strong by lowering your blood pressure and improving your cholesterol profile.

> Strength training can help decrease PMS symptoms associated with monthly hormone fluctuations.

> Strength training can reverse certain aging factors in skeletal muscle and can protect against oxidative cell damage that can lead to diseases of aging, like cancer and diabetes.

> Strength training can reduce stress, improve your sleep, and pump up your confidence and self-worth, which will go a long way toward easing symptoms of depression, if you're suffering, and enhancing your overall mental health.

That's a boatload of body benefits, if you ask me. Who wouldn't want all of that? You certainly deserve it. And you'll get it all—if you Lift to Get Lean.

Holly Perkins

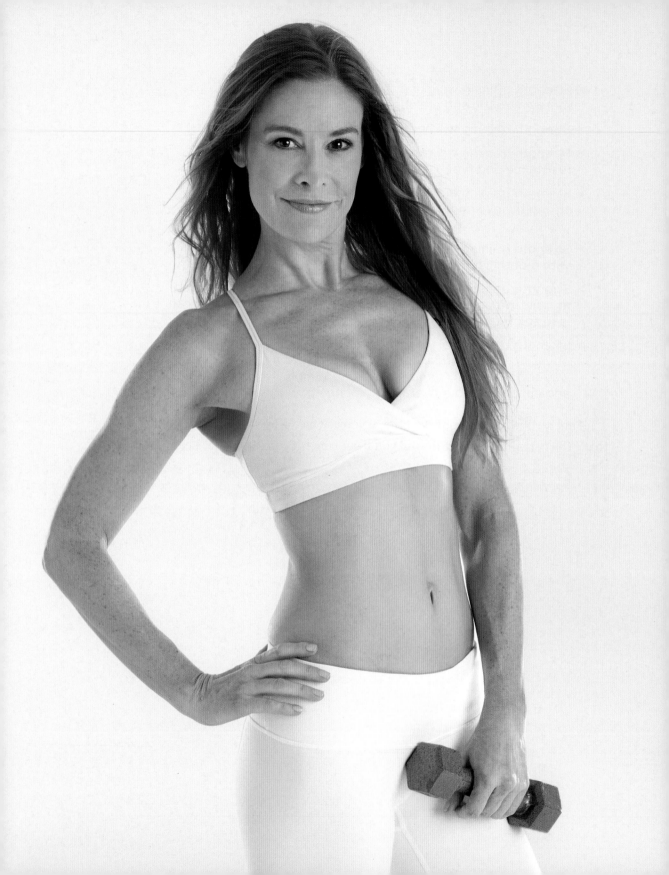

Part I
The Foundation

Lift to Get Lean

Chapter 1
Lift Like a Girl!

I am not a man. You are not a man. So why do we exercise like men do? It bears repeating: We've been taught to train like men because weight lifting has always been the domain of male athletes and male-dominated sports. It was that way when I started out in the fitness business more than 20 years ago.

Let me tell you my story and how I came to the realization that there must be a better way for women to get lean and strong.

After I graduated from Penn State, I was offered a job at a prestigious health and fitness facility in New York City as an exercise physiologist and personal trainer. The facility was owned and operated by a very successful personal trainer to Madonna, Julia Roberts, Howard Stern, and numerous other A-listers. At the time, he was *the* person to train with and learn from. He became my mentor (and boss) and gave me my foundation. Although he was a great mentor, he was a guy, and he handed down all of the rules of weight lifting from a man's perspective, including the original bro exercises—the classic, go-to exercises that the boys have taught us women to do. They are exercises that work great for them but not for a woman's body. This is one example why women have been learning strength training wrong all along—we have always learned from the guys. Guys teach what guys know and what works for their bodies. It's an industry led by men. But now you are going to start doing things the right way. Our way.

I came out of college certain that I knew everything there was to know about crafting supreme health and fitness programs for my clients and myself. I had extensive knowledge about physiology, nutrition, biomechanics, energy production, muscle development, and cardiovascular fitness. I knew it all! I exploded out of the gates and into New York City to begin my career as a personal trainer and coach. I spent almost 3 years consumed with fitness and arrived at age 25 exhausted, clinically depressed, plagued by debilitating pain in both knees, dependent on caffeine, controlled by sugar cravings, severely sleep deprived, constipated, and really cranky. If you knew me during this time in my life, please accept my apologies!

The worst part of it all was that I thought these issues were part of the trade-off for looking fit. I was doing 60 to 90 minutes of cardio every day. I would go into the weight room and do a few exercises, but I wasn't following a program. And when I did lift weights, I would go heavy—in retrospect, far too heavy for my skill level at the time.

But even with all that effort, I still didn't look fit! My body fat was around 28 percent; I was at least 15 pounds overweight and had serious muscle imbalances because I had no strength.

I distinctly remember one morning when I was doing everything in my power to drum up enough energy to get out the door and into Central Park for a run. I had created a list of things that I could do on the days when I was crippled with fatigue and needed to force my body into a workout. I called this my "Big Guns" list because it included things that I wouldn't normally do before a workout.

On this day, I had four shots of espresso, two Advil, and two ephedra capsules (this was before ephedra was taken off the market because it's so dangerous), and I taped both of my knees in hopes of some pain relief. Because the fitness experts at the time said I would burn more body fat if I did cardio on an empty stomach, I hadn't eaten breakfast. (Please don't try this at home!) Despite these powerful Big Guns, I was wrecked and could not get myself out the door. I had hit a wall. I mean, I had hit a 20-foot cement roadblock. All of a sudden, I realized how badly I felt on a very deep physical, spiritual, and mental level. I felt physically ill despite doing everything that I thought I was supposed to do. Every nook of my body hurt, and I was lying flat-out on the floor.

I remember thinking, "I have a BS in exercise physiology with an emphasis in nutrition. I have high-level certifications and work at the most prestigious gym in the world with the most famous celebrities ever. How is it possible that I can feel so lost, totally overwhelmed, and completely confused about my health and fitness? If I'm confused, how on earth are average folks supposed to figure it out?"

My Turning Point

Then a moment came where I simultaneously felt more desperation than I had ever experienced and an equally deep sense of calm and pure presence. I had hit rock bottom. It was a feeling of complete loss of control—and beauty. The only way left to go was up, and I had no choice but to go. In that moment, I felt a clear sense of resolve. I *had* to figure this out. My magical guru didn't show up, so I set out to become my own guru.

I spent the next 10 years exploring and evaluating every workout and diet on the market. I read every major book, pored over research articles, and attended conferences. If I wasn't comfortable testing out a system on a client, I would use myself as a guinea pig. I worked with doctors, physical therapists, nutritionists, and psychologists. One baby step at a time, I sorted through the trends to find the systems that resonated with me and produced the desired results. I was on a mission; I felt an extreme sense of purpose, and it energized me.

Research shows that the best way to make true, permanent habit changes is through small, consistent lifestyle changes. Many, many lifestyle changes later— like 15 years of baby steps later—I was approaching my 40th birthday feeling pretty good. But then a perfect storm of sorts came one day, and I found myself at an emotional rock bottom again. The big 4-0 was near, my marriage was ending, my beloved dog was dying, and I felt completely alone. Have you ever experienced a flood of disappointments like this? I think we all have at some point. It caused me to take a hard look at myself again: I had spent my entire career in fitness, and I was absolutely not the image of empowerment and well-being that I wanted to be.

At that moment, another seed of resolve sprouted, and once again I felt there was nowhere to go but up. It was time to start climbing again.

A New Fit and Empowered Self

At that point, I had tried every fitness workout, plan, and strategy in existence—except one. I had never trained with the goal of making my body stronger. Sure, I would lift weights—go into the weight room, do a few bro exercises—but I had never trained for strength in the way that one would train for a 5-K or any other fitness goal. It was my last option, so I took it.

Part of me knew that the only way I would survive the emotional battle of my personal life was by building a supremely strong physical life. It was as though I knew that through strength training I would find emotional strength. Lifting weights to create my dream body would also create personal strength. This is why I now choose to say "strength training."

I scheduled a photo shoot to keep myself accountable. It took me about a year to truly transform my body. In an oddly perfect sort of way, that year was absolutely the most challenging year of my entire life. I had set out to remodel my body and ended up reprogramming my whole life on a physical, emotional, mental, and spiritual level.

The gym became my metaphor for life. My commitment to bettering my body forced me to work through the tough times. Those tough times made me examine my motivations, my defense mechanisms, and the excuses that I had been allowing myself to make. I had been beaten down emotionally, and strength training built me back up. As I strengthened my body, I rebuilt my life. I had successfully broken my sugar and caffeine dependency, healed my knees naturally, optimized my digestion, improved my mental health, and started experiencing days where I felt sooooo good, almost euphoric. It made me realize how terrible I had been feeling nearly my whole adult life. And I started to cry.

The Power of Strength Training for Women

I emerged reborn at 42. I was a new woman with a new perspective on life, a deep and unshakable sense of strength, and a system of training that works best for the female body. I have more energy now, at 42, than I had in my twenties. I am leaner and more fit and functional than I was in my thirties. And when I get compliments, I hear, "You look amazing," not "You look amazing for your age." I don't say this to brag. I say this as a testament to the power of strength training. I say this because you are no different than I—regardless of your age—and I want this for you as well. I say this because I know that you can achieve the very same thing for yourself and that it will change your life, too.

Mine was a wonderful journey through a million little baby steps. Yours begins now, and it'll be a much shorter trip. I promise.

Chapter 2
The Secret to Getting Lean for Life

I've noticed an interesting pattern with my female clients over the years. When I ask their exact reasons for coming to me, the most common response is that they want to look better. Immediately after telling me this, they look embarrassed and some of them comment on how they feel vain for saying that. As I dig into this with them, they reveal that they believe society views vanity as a shallow and negative motivator and that they shouldn't be concerned with their looks. It's as though they feel ashamed for wanting to look better!

Here's a very important fact to accept: It's perfectly human to want to feel good about how you look. You should feel proud of yourself for wanting to take care of your appearance, because doing so is a sign of self-respect. Own your vanity and wear it with pride. I applaud you for being brave enough to say: "I want to look better and I'm going to." Honor the part of you that wants this for yourself, even if it isn't your primary motivator.

At the same time, simply looking good for others is never going to be enough to motivate you to make a true, radical, and lasting change. If it was enough, well, you'd probably have your ideal body already and you wouldn't need this book!

The Three Most Common Lies Women Tell Themselves

So why haven't you achieved your personal vision of fitness yet? I've had this conversation countless times. And I believe the reason most women haven't achieved their best bodies is twofold.

1. They don't know how to accomplish it because they haven't found a system that works.
2. They think they are motivated purely by vanity and that bothers them.

But when I ask women why they don't have their dream bodies, they usually respond in one of three ways.

> "I'm lazy."
> "I must not want it bad enough."
> "My body is 'quirky' and doesn't seem to respond well to exercise."

Let's take a look at these beliefs one by one.

"I'm lazy."

If you were to look at all the areas of your life, would you say that you are a lazy person? Do you work hard? Is there something in your life that you kick butt at? If so, you are not lazy. You might have some motivation problems around fitness, but you are not lazy. Going forward, give yourself a break from playing the laziness card. Laziness is not your problem.

"I must not want it bad enough."

When you think about having a rockin' bod, do you get excited? Does it spark something big and expansive inside of you? Do you feel a powerful kind of energy when you visualize it? Then you *do* want it enough. You just don't know how to get it without crazy-hard workouts, hours of cardio, or a diet that turns you into a hangry (hungry + angry) grump monster. I bet you want your dream body a lot; you just don't know how to achieve it. Yet.

"My body is 'quirky' and doesn't seem to respond well to exercise."

Have you ever had a moment in your life when you were really happy with your body or fitness level? Was there ever a time when you followed a diet or fitness plan and saw results? If so, this is proof that your body is perfectly equipped to respond to your diet and fitness efforts. You're not as quirky as you think! You've done it before, and you can do it again.

If you have never seen progress from following a diet or fitness plan, it's possible that you haven't found a system that's right for your body. Or perhaps you haven't found the right motivations, so you drop a program before it can have a noticeable effect. Or maybe you feared bulking up and dialed way back just when you should have kept pushing.

In the chapters to come, you'll learn the solutions to all of these challenges. And because everyone is different, you'll also learn how to discover the solutions that work for you.

You *can* influence the state of your body. You *do* have the ability to create the body of your dreams. It is absolutely possible for you to lift and get lean.

You *can* influence the state of your body. You *do* have the ability to create the body of your dreams. It is absolutely possible for you to lift and get lean.

Why Some People Succeed—
And How to Crib Their Secret

While my degree is in exercise physiology, not psychology, I do know what makes people successful at achieving their ideal bodies. **The reason why some people have achieved their dream bodies is because they are connected to their truest motivations.** Yes, for some people, that motivation is vanity. But for many others—myself included—it is a reflection of the standard to which we hold ourselves. It is a demonstration of the respect we have for our bodies. It is the belief that our bodies are a gift and it is our duty to maximize their potential. We do it because it's who we are, it's how we become better, and it's how we express our life force.

I was able to change my life and achieve a superior level of fitness because I finally came to understand that I am worthy of achieving something that I want for myself. Self-worth does not come from a lifted butt, perky breasts, or a flat stomach. Your self-worth is the value you hold for yourself that is inherent and deep inside. It is present throughout all of your decisions and experiences. It is what allows you to go after your dreams.

For years I thought that successful people had something special that I did not have. I thought they had been blessed with some magical traits that I had been deprived of. I thought that their ability to be exceptional came easily because they were born with superpowers. They just had more energy or were smarter or more intuitive. I had to realize that I, too, am worthy of such greatness. Those people didn't have any magical traits that I didn't have. Exceptional people are exceptional because they believe they are worthy of greatness and capable of achieving it and because they take massive action.

In other words, they create their own superpowers. And you can, too.

Exceptional people are exceptional because they _believe_ they are worthy of greatness and _capable_ of achieving it and because they take massive action.

The Achievement Mind-Set

One of the biggest myths in health and fitness is that body transformation is easy. Despite what many headlines and advertisements tell you, creating real change and becoming fit is actually a bit challenging. If it were easy, everyone would be superfit, right?

Getting fit requires discipline, commitment, and consistency. I have found that it is these human factors that make fitness gains the most difficult—not laziness or lack of desire. At times, getting fit requires you to dig deep when you are tired, push when you don't want to, and step up when you'd rather lie down.

This is why vanity is not an effective motivator for most people and why it's imperative that you are connected to bigger motivators. When the day comes (and it will) that you are supposed to hit the gym for a workout but you're not in the mood, you'll think, "Meh. I can skip the gym today. I'm an awesome person

Yes, You Can Do This!

My clients tell me that the reason they finally succeeded in changing their bodies was because I told them that it was possible. I realize that I have never seen your body. But I will tell you this now with 100 percent certainty: It *is* possible to achieve the body that you want. I promise you. On the days when you doubt yourself, rely on my belief in you. Trust in my faith in your abilities and you will see incredible results. Whatever you want for yourself, trust me, it's possible.

I have a motto when I start working with new clients, "If you do what I tell you to do, you will get tremendous results." Problems set in when my clients aren't able or willing to integrate the actions that I suggest. There really is truth in the saying: "When the student is ready, the teacher will appear." Once a client is truly ready for change, she hears everything I say and takes massive action. That's when all the good stuff starts to happen. You must *do* in order to *get!*

no matter what I look like." Your vanity goes out the window when you're tired, stressed, or pressed for time. In order to overcome these obstacles and create the body of your dreams, you must be connected to more powerful motivations. You must be motivated by your higher self.

Our superpowers come from achievement. They come from overcoming obstacles and hardships. It is the essence of the human spirit. Resilience is built only after you've stayed committed to something despite its difficulty. We grow and become better through challenge. And we experience thrill, victory, and joy when we accomplish something that we weren't sure we could. Through this quest for personal excellence, we develop our superpowers.

Rock-solid empowerment and unshakable self-respect come from digging deep, working hard, and sticking to your guns—even when you don't feel like it. And that will be far easier if you are motivated by something much bigger than looks alone.

Only by cultivating your best "you" can you create your best body.

Commit to Yourself

It helps to identify your motivators, but at the end of the day, creating a lean body just comes down to *doing it*. You literally just have to take action—massive action. An object in motion tends to stay in motion. An object at rest tends to stay at rest. You've got to get moving, override inertia, and make this happen for yourself.

Each day, I want you to connect with a deep and true part of yourself. I want you to feel the thrill that will occur in 90 days when you discover that you have cultivated a strong, resilient, and empowered self. This part of you is responsible for creating a body that reflects your inner excellence.

So let's agree on the following:

1. You are *not* lazy.
2. You *do* want it bad enough.
3. You *believe* that your body truly has the potential to blossom into something strong, powerful, and fantastic.

This book will take you on a journey in the gym to cultivate a deeper sense of you. Changing your body will change you in so many incredible ways. If you commit 100 percent to following one of the Lift to Get Lean 90-day programs (Chapters 9 to 12), you will emerge with a powerful sense of achievement, resilience, and both physical and personal strength. These are the things that the human spirit most truly desires. A slammin' bod is just something that comes as a result of these other things. Creating a lean, buff body is a piece of cake when you approach it this way. But hear me clearly: The only way to these rewards is through massive action.

Our superpowers come from *achievement*. They come from overcoming obstacles and hardships. It is the *essence* of the human spirit.

Chapter 3
A New System Designed Precisely for Women

I hope I've started to convince you that when it comes to strength training, what works for men does not work for women. We are drastically in need of a new plan created for a woman's body, psychology, and hormones. And you have it right here.

My dream is to educate you on the facts of proper strength training so that you will become inspired to walk confidently into the weights section of your gym and begin your journey. Before we get started, let's take a look at eight key principles that will help you build a strong body.

The Plan: A Selfie of Your Journey

1. **Do one program for 90 days.** Now, 3 months may seem like a long time, but think of it this way: You're adopting a new

lifestyle, and strength training will become an integral part of it. This isn't something you do for a couple of weeks, stop, and then go back to living the same old way. Meaningful change doesn't happen like that. Do one 90-day program and I guarantee you'll be hooked and eager to try another.

2. **Join a gym if you don't already belong to one.** In order to do all the exercises in the Lift to Get Lean 90-day training programs that start in Chapter 9, you need to have access to a gym or health club. I made a very conscious decision to create these workouts to be done in a traditional gym setting. Why? My goal is to help you cultivate a new kind of strength that you most likely have not experienced yet. The most effective path to a lean, strong, feminine look is through a very specific kind of strength training called progressive resistance (challenging your muscles more and more over time). Research shows that it is critical to increasing strength and lean muscle mass. But progressive resistance training requires specialized equipment that typically only exists in gyms. You need a variety of weights, cables, bars, and pulleys, as well as exercise machines with different weight loads to achieve the lean look you want. It is possible to get lean in a home gym, but there will inevitably be compromises made that will limit and slow your progress. Take the Leg Curl exercise, for example. I have yet to meet a home version of a leg curl machine that actually loads the muscle in the ideal way. The leg curl machine at your local gym is going to be your best friend for creating incredible hamstrings. Once you see the results, you'll be singing the praises of gym life along with me. Another movement that is nearly impossible to do effectively at home is the Reverse Grip Pulldown. Again, unless you have a very expensive, very extensive home gym, you will miss out on this critical exercise. The Reverse Grip Pulldown is the most important movement for your entire upper body. It is critical for optimal posture, alignment, spine stability, and pulling strength. In my practice, the most common reason for shoulder problems is insufficient

pulling strength. Pretty much the only way to hit these important back muscles effectively is through the Reverse Grip Pulldown movement.

I realize that it might be inconvenient to join a gym. Or maybe you are avoiding the gym because you are nervous about the unfamiliar environment or intimidated by it. If you are still a bit reluctant to join a gym, I encourage you to honestly examine your reasons and consider them against the changes that you want to see in your body.

3. **Understand how your muscles and body work.** You will get faster results in the gym if you are able to fully comprehend the systems that are at play when you exercise. Think of this as the ultimate mind-body connection. For example, a basic principle in developing lean muscle through progressive resistance is called *overload*. It simply means that in order to create new change in a muscle, you must challenge it beyond its current ability and continue to do that progressively over time. However, there is an interesting survival mechanism that kicks in when you do something beyond your current ability, and it can limit your progress if you are not aware of how it works. Learn how to override this mechanism (plus plenty of other goodies) in Chapter 5.

4. **Follow my Three-Step System to Strength.** Every month, popular magazines and Web sites interview me about my favorite exercises for various body parts. I find that to be backward thinking, though. They put so much emphasis on exercise selection and very little on exercise execution. The latter—how you perform the movements and sets—is the most critical part of effective strength training. In order to create beautifully sculpted, feminine muscles that are balanced and proportionate, you must perform the exercises using a very specific technique. In Chapter 6, you'll learn exactly how to perform any strength-training exercise so that it will give you the best results. This is the most critical part of strength workouts because it makes any movement effective. It is my

secret sauce to getting strong and lean. First get your technique down, that's step one, and then learn the two tricks that will ensure you get the most from every workout.

5. **Perform the right exercises to create curves where you want them.** I don't know about you, but I want very different curves and muscle definition than my hunky guy. A big, thick chest and wide cobra back are sexy on a man, but most women want something different. There is a handful of exercises that work great for men but aren't so great for women. I have found a set of key exercises that work best for a woman's body, and I've

"Women Can't Bulk Up": True or False?

There is a great deal of confusion in the fitness industry right now about whether women can "bulk up" or not. The truth is that every woman has the ability to increase the size of her muscles to some degree. However, because of hormonal influences, most women aren't able to build muscle to the degree that men can.

Now, some women are more inclined to develop muscle size. But even for these women, building muscle bulk requires a great deal of long-term effort. In fact, at different times in my career, I have intentionally used some bro exercises so that I could beef up my frame. It took a ton of effort, highly strategic eating, and a traditional male bodybuilding workout plan.

When I was filming for my home workout system, called baladea, I wanted a very feminine physique. So I used the exercises and workout plan in this book to create a lean, but softer, look.

The vast majority of women are interested in building a lean, feminine body that appears toned rather than muscular. And in my experience, 90 percent of women do not have the hormonal profile or the desire to build a substantial amount of muscle.

My point is that, yes, women can bulk up if they choose to, but it takes a massive amount of intention, and it certainly does not happen within 90 days of strength training.

also identified the exercises that many women should avoid in order to create the most feminine frame. In Chapter 7, you'll learn the exercises that work best for women through simple step-by-step descriptions and photos.

6. **Choose moves that will add definition, not size.** The exercises and workouts in this book have been chosen with great care to strategically build you the most attractive body without much increase in muscle size. Sometimes all it takes is a hand position

Let's Talk about "Gym-Timidation"

I still remember the very first time I walked into the weights section of my gym at Pennsylvania State University. Back then, many institutions had separate weight rooms just for women, and Penn State had one for students and staff. It was a small room with old equipment, poor lighting, and no music. Basically, no "love." I remember staring at the seated leg curl machine in complete horror. I had no idea what to do with it. I knew it was for the hamstrings, but I honestly had no idea how to manipulate the machine to adjust the seat and leg levers. It was a scary contraption and I felt intimidated by it, so I walked out.

That day was a major buzzkill, and it took me a year to take another stab at it. This time, I went to the coed facility so that I could learn by watching the boys and have access to better equipment. But there was a new terror—men. This time I really felt intimidated because I knew the men were watching me. I felt like an alien! I was so awkward and confused.

It took many more years for me to get comfortable in the weights section of the gym and find my groove. Now when I see a woman like me venturing into the weights section for the first time, my heart swells and pounds. I want to run over and squeeze her and say, "You can do this! Come play with me!" And this is exactly what I get to do for you in this book. We'll walk through a day in the weight room together so you'll feel confident and excited. We're going to make the weight room your happy place.

change to make a bro exercise perfect for a woman. All exercises have variations to accentuate different body areas. For example, there is a specific back exercise that will make your biceps look *ahhh-mazing*. And it works better than many traditional biceps exercises. (Find out what it is on page 76.) Chapter 7 will walk you through all of my favorite movements that create the lean and feminine physique that you want, without adding bulk. And if you happen to be one of the 10 percent of women who *do* want to increase muscle mass, I have a 90-day training program for you, too (see page 149)!

7. **Follow the right plan for you.** Are you a beginner? Or are you already a regular in the gym? There are four amazing 90-day training programs in this book. Each is designed for a different fitness level and body type. Most likely, one of my programs will resonate with you immediately, and you'll know it's the right one for you. I will ask you some questions to direct you to the right program if you are still unsure. And I'll walk you through a sample workout step-by-step so you'll feel totally confident. You'll know exactly what to do, when to do it, and how to navigate the sometimes-confusing gym playground. Once you finish with one program, you can try another!

8. **Cultivate a fit lifestyle.** What your body looks like comes down to three broad areas: strength training, cardio, and lifestyle habits. While the emphasis of this book is on strength training, I will also give you some tips on incorporating cardio into the program and little tricks to improve your diet and sleep habits, all of which will boost your fitness progress. But you will find that improvements in lifestyle habits come naturally once you develop a routine of strength training and start seeing results. Cardio will be something to round out your program for health and general fitness. You will soon understand that it is only through consistent strength training that you'll remodel your musculature and rewire your metabolism to create the body you've always wanted. In order to get lean, you must get strong.

Chapter 4
Why Strength Training Matters to Your Health

You've admired, even envied, the arms of women rocking sleeveless shirts and strapless dresses. Or maybe you're looking to tone up your legs, sculpt a booty-shorts-worthy backside, or squeeze into your favorite skinny jeans again. Whatever your motivation, strength training is your secret weapon to the kind of body you've always wanted. But the benefits working out with weights delivers go far beyond vanity. While you're working out to look slimmer, stronger, and sexier, you'll also be taking action toward building greater overall health and a rock-solid self-esteem.

Strength training is critically important to your health. It's as important as choosing not to smoke, eating healthy whole foods, going for an annual doctor's visit, and flossing your teeth. It's something you'll want to make a part of your lifestyle permanently, not just for a month before the start of bikini season. So let's take a closer look at what strength training can do for you on every level.

You'll want to reread this chapter whenever you get the urge to skip a workout. You simply don't want to cheat your body out of any of this good stuff!

Weight Loss That Stays Off

Building lean muscle is the most effective way to lower your body fat and stay trim for life. To understand how muscle works its magic, it helps to know a little about the tissue itself. For one, it's more densely packed than fat; flab takes up about 18 percent more space on your body. So the more muscle you have, the leaner your body will look simply because it's more compact. The second reason more muscle is better for weight loss: Muscle is more metabolically active than fat. In other words, it requires significantly more calories of energy to maintain than fat does. So more muscle means more calorie burn around the clock. Strength training, therefore, offers a double-barreled benefit for trimming down, which was apparent in a study published by the American College of Sports Medicine. The study showed that women who strength trained two to three times a week gained 2 pounds of lean muscle and lost 3.5 pounds of fat over the course of just 2 months.

A Decrease in Belly Fat

Strength training is becoming increasingly important in the war against obesity as researchers continue to show evidence of resistance exercise's powerful impact on fat reduction, particularly in the abdominal region. Studies of women who have taken up strength training show a reduction of intra-abdominal fat (the most dangerous fat, which forms around your abdominal organs). What's more, research suggests that regular strength training can help women avoid weight gain as they get older. In a study at the University of Minnesota, two groups of overweight women were monitored for 2 years. Those women who did twice-weekly strength-training routines of 10 exercises targeting the major muscle groups gained 67 percent less abdominal fat than another group of sedentary women who did not strength train.

A Faster Metabolism

Building more lean muscle mass delivers a dual impact on the number of calories you burn while doing nothing, what's referred to as your resting metabolism. First, as you've already learned, more muscle requires more energy for simple tissue maintenance. Second, every time you strength train, your workout causes microtraumas, or tiny tears, throughout your muscle tissue that require lots of energy for repair and rebuilding. Studies by Wayne Westcott, PhD, of the American College of Sports Medicine found resistance training stimulates increased muscle protein turnover, elevating the resting metabolic rate of beginners by an average of 5 percent for 3 full days after a weight-lifting workout. Westcott's research suggests that strength training regularly may boost your resting metabolic rate by up to 9 percent, enough to burn 100 extra calories per day!

Cardio-only workouts burn calories initially while you are working out, but they don't deliver the kind of afterburn that strength training does. In my experience (and that of many of the women I train) cardio-only workouts can actually backfire, tricking you into thinking you're burning more calories than you really are and making you hungrier, which may lead you to munch more calories than your exercise eliminated.

A Younger Body

After age 30, everyone starts to lose 3 to 8 percent of her muscle mass every 10 years, and that percentage increases to as much as 10 percent starting in the fifth decade of life. No wonder we put on weight as we age. A study in the *American Journal of Clinical Nutrition* found that for every pound of muscle a person loses, she will typically gain a pound of fat!

The type of muscle we lose plays a significant role in how quickly we show the signs of aging. There are two types of muscle fibers—fast-twitch and slow-twitch. Slow-twitch muscles are responsible for endurance and fast-twitch for generating power. We lose significantly more fast-twitch muscle fibers as we age, which is important to know because fast-twitch muscles are the ones we need for sports performance and for pushing ourselves out of a chair. Fast-twitch are known as the longevity muscle fibers; you need them to stay strong and active as you age. So how do we save them? By using powerful movements during strength-training workouts. In Chapter 6, you'll learn my secret to firing up those important muscle fibers and ensuring a mega metabolic boost.

Stronger Bones

Stressing your bones by doing weight-bearing exercises instructs your body to lay down new bone, strengthening your skeleton. If you aren't lifting weights, you're missing out on a key natural strategy to boost your bone mineral density and prevent osteoporosis, a progressive bone disease affecting nearly 8 million women, according to the National Osteoporosis Foundation. Studies reported in the *Journal of Bone and Mineral Research* show that resistance training increases bone mineral density by 1 to 3 percent in pre- and postmenopausal women.

A Reduced Risk of Diabetes

According to the American Diabetes Association, 86 million Americans over the age of 20 have prediabetes, the precursor to full-blown type 2 diabetes, the deadly disease that experts believe will affect one out of every three adults by the middle of this century. Research has shown that strength training can improve your body's ability to use the hormone insulin to effectively clear glucose (sugar) from your bloodstream.

One study published in the journal *Diabetes* reported that both men and women became more insulin sensitive after 12 weeks of strength training. Greater insulin sensitivity allows your body to better regulate the amount of glucose in your bloodstream to combat cravings for sugar, balance your energy levels, and reduce the accumulation of belly fat. One recent study that looked specifically at women and exercise found that strength training for at least 1 hour a week slashed a woman's risk of developing type 2 diabetes by 28 percent. All of the workouts in this book ensure that you'll be meeting that minimum.

A Stronger Heart

It tells you something when the American Heart Association starts recommending strength training as therapy for patients in cardiac rehabilitation programs. The research clearly shows that strength training is an important weapon against heart disease, which kills one in four women in the United States, according to reports from the National Institutes of Health.

A study by the American College of Sports Medicine found that a combination of strength and aerobic training reduces blood pressure and body fat, improves cholesterol profiles, and even keeps blood vessels pliable. In similar research, the *Journal of Strength and Conditioning Research* reported on a study that showed women who lifted weights were 37 percent less likely to have metabolic syndrome, a cluster of conditions that contributes to weight gain and increases your risk of heart disease.

Improved Mood

Balance your hormones each time you pick up a barbell. Strength training has been associated with a substantial decrease in monthly hormone fluctuations. Weight training reduces cortisol, a stress hormone in your bloodstream that quickens your heartbeat, feeds your brain extra oxygen, and unleashes energy from fat and glucose. While elevated cortisol levels can be good in a pinch, tapping your cortisol bank can cause unrelenting stress and leave you feeling tired. Incorporating resistance training and short bouts of cardio will better manage your cortisol levels to prevent spikes that leave you feeling spent.

Similarly, testosterone plays a crucial role in your energy levels and hormone balance. Too little can leave you feeling sluggish, depressed, and disinterested in your significant other. Lifting weights lights up natural testosterone levels in your body, which can improve your sex drive, muscle strength, bone density, and metabolism. Improving your mood could be beneficial to your career, too. Research published in the *Journal of Occupational and Environmental Medicine* found that workers were 15 percent more productive on days they made time to exercise, and they were 15 percent more tolerant of their coworkers.

Less Pain

Osteoarthritis causes inflammation and pain around your joints due to the wearing away of cartilage. Strength training makes the muscles around those painful joints stronger, allowing them to better support the joints, which takes away some of the pressure and eases the pain. In one study, elderly folks with severe knee osteoarthritis decreased their pain by an average of 43 percent during a 16-week strength-training program. But don't wait until you've got grandkids to start doing squats. Combined with daily stretching, strength training can prevent the atrophy of joint cartilage, so you can keep skiing the bumps in your seventies. Even if you don't have full-blown osteoarthritis, strength training can alleviate many general aches and pains. Stronger muscles mean better alignment of all of your joints.

Easier Crossword Puzzles

Lifting weights can even make your brain buff. In one study, Brazilian researchers found that 6 months of strength training resulted in improvements in markers of cognitive health, such as short- and long-term memory, attention span, and scores on verbal reasoning tests.

Better Sleep Quality

You don't need a scientist to tell you that rigorous exercise will cue your body for more restful sleep. You've probably felt it happen in your own life. But for people who suffer from debilitating sleep disorders, regular strength training could be their drug-free ticket to a good night's sleep. In one study, depressed people with sleep disorders showed a 30 percent improvement in sleep after 8 weeks of regular strength training.

Greater Confidence and Self-Esteem

Strength training changed my life. It boosted my self-esteem during times of difficulty, and I've seen it happen in my clients, too. Making your muscles stronger also makes your resolve to do better in all aspects of your life stronger. It makes you feel good about your body and leaves you with a satisfying sense of accomplishment. It's no wonder the research shows that exercising regularly with weights delivers significant mental health benefits, including reductions in symptoms of depression, anxiety, and fatigue. Strength training also has been shown to help women feel better about their bodies and appearance, according to research published in the *New England Journal of Medicine.* In a 12-month study, researchers at the University of Pennsylvania School of Medicine tested the impact of twice-weekly weight-lifting sessions on breast cancer survivors' physical and emotional health. They found that the breast cancer survivors who strength trained twice a week saw a 12 percent improvement in their body images and satisfaction with their intimate relationships, compared with just a 2 percent improvement for women who didn't lift weights.

· · · · ·

An interesting thing happens as you progress through the 90-day training programs in this book: You will see many of your health problems diminish. As your sleep improves and your fatigue subsides, you will find you have more energy and willpower to direct toward your workouts and diet choices. As you add muscle to your frame, you'll notice the weight coming off quicker, and that positive, measurable feedback will encourage you to stick to your healthy eating plan. As you lose weight, you may find that your joints ache less and there's a new pep in your step. You'll start to feel more confident, less stressed, happier.

You've heard of the mind-body connection. Well, I like to think of it as the body-mind connection, because your body chemicals influence your mind and emotions. When good things are happening in your body, your brain benefits. Your entire system functions optimally.

Many of us consider living disease-free as the definition of healthy. Not me. That's not good enough. I want to live a life that is vibrant, exuberant, and thriving. I want to feel boundless in my energy and life spirit. I want to run, jump, and play with physical enthusiasm every day for the rest of my life. And I know you do, too. Strength training will help you shed your health burdens and live the life you deserve in the body you want.

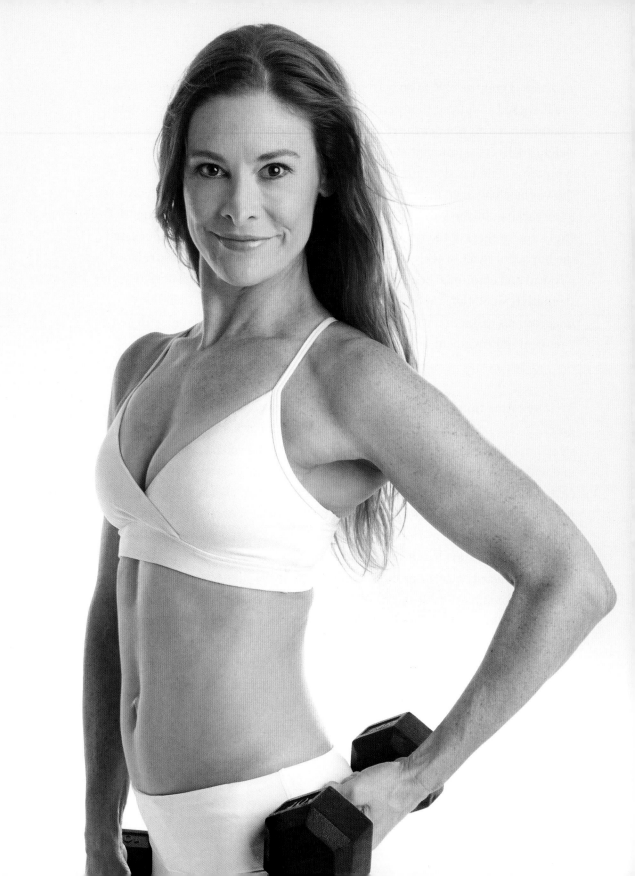

Part II
Systems and Movements

Lift
to Get
Lean

Chapter 5
How to Make a Muscle (And Why It's So Hard to Change)

You may be only 45 or 31 or even 23, but your body is ancient. Behaviorally, we humans may have made great strides, but anatomically our bodies are very much like those of our hairier ancestors some 200,000 years ago.

Anthropologists say that our bodies evolved in ways that ensure our survival in a constantly changing environment. We have built-in systems designed for homeostasis that keep our bodies on an even keel—happy and cozy and unchanging.

Think about it. Appetite occurs when you need calories to maintain your body size and energy needs. Fatigue happens when you need sleep so that your body can be restored and revitalized. You start to shiver when the biting cold threatens your 98.6-degree internal temperature, and blood moves out of your extremities inward to protect your vital organs. Your heart rate increases, your eyes widen, and blood shoots to your arms and legs to fuel action when you feel threatened. All of these responses are your body's automatic attempts to deal with crisis and return to homeostasis. To put it simply, your body abhors change and will do anything in its power to return to a state of safety and boring sameness. It sees any change as a threat and fights hard for homeostasis, even when change would be good for you. That's one reason losing weight and gaining muscle strength are so difficult to accomplish. Your body doesn't want to go there—even after reading about all those benefits in Chapter 4!

Outsmart Evolution

In order to create a change in your body, you must override your current scenario—your homeostasis—and that usually requires actions that are different from what you've been doing. In order to change, *you* must change. You need to break out of your comfort zone. This is why I relate muscular growth in the gym to personal growth in your life. It's all the same! You have to be uncomfortable if you want to achieve something bigger and better.

The only way to override homeostasis and create change is to expose your body to the new stimulus over and over and over. In training for strength, that means exposing your muscles to progressive resistance, heavier and heavier weights that keep on challenging them. In essence, you need to make your muscles work harder and harder. There's no way to sugarcoat this. The exercises don't get easier, but you will get better.

All of the 90-day training programs in this book are designed around this concept and provide your muscles with the perfect amount of "stress" to make them stronger. Each month, your program will progress so that you are tackling new challenges and pushing your muscles to break through homeostasis. Each month, the workout will get harder, and you will get stronger, leaner, and fitter. Remember, a pound of muscle is smaller in size than a pound of fat, so even if the weight on the scale doesn't change (and it will), you are going to be smaller and tighter if you add muscle.

Take *that,* ancient body!

Your Body on Strength Training

In the gym you create muscle and strength by exposing your body to resistance that is beyond your current ability. Over time, continued exposure forces your muscles to physically change. The technical term for this is *hypertrophy*. When a muscle is significantly challenged, muscle cells become agitated, kicking off a chain reaction that increases the diameter of the muscle fiber. The amount of challenge you put on your muscle can be called tension. Maybe you've heard the phrase "time under tension." It's a very important concept in strength training. Lifting a light object causes a small amount of tension. Lifting a heavy object slowly causes great tension. This is where the magic happens. Heavy tension causes microscopic tears in your muscle fibers. The greater the pressure inside your muscle, the more extensive the "damage" to your muscle fibers. But I don't want you to think of this damage as a bad thing because it's ultimately what helps you become stronger.

Damage is the building block of strength and muscle development. The greater the time and pressure, the greater the damage to your muscle. This breaking down is followed by a period of repair and recovery. This is the special sauce where the real strength and muscles are made. Your workouts are only as good as your recoveries.

Here are the changes that you can expect to happen to your body by following the 90-day programs toward the end of this book.

It doesn't get *easier*. You get *better*.

The First 4 Weeks: You'll Get Superstrong

Long before your muscle size changes, you will notice considerable improvements in strength. What's happening here has to do with neuromuscular changes—changes in the neurons and other brain structures that activate your muscles. When you intend to move a muscle, your brain must first send a signal down your spinal cord to a motor neuron. That signal is what makes your muscle fire. You must first think, then you'll move.

When you first start strength training, your ability to call your motor neurons into action is limited. And because you're not using all of your motor neurons, you're not using all of your muscle fibers, which limits your strength. Weak muscles are simply "sleepy" muscles, and we need to wake 'em up!

Tips for Speedier Strength Gains

The real boost from strength training comes after you leave the gym and your body starts the repair and recovery process. Here are some ways you can speed this up.

1. Eat a small meal or snack as soon as you can after your workout. Make it a combination of fast-digesting protein and carbohydrates. Try some chocolate whey protein powder stirred into milk, dates with some banana and nut butter, or an apple and string cheese.

2. Be sure to eat something every 3 to 4 hours after your workouts. Eat meals and snacks containing a balance of protein, fat, and carbohydrates.

3. Stay active during the days in between your strength workouts. Active recovery improves bloodflow, which promotes healing. Taking a brisk walk or a casual bike ride, foam rolling, or just splashing around in a pool are all good options.

4. Find some stress management tools that work for you. The stress hormone cortisol is catabolic, meaning it eats away at muscle and strength. Protect your hard-earned strength by de-stressing with mindful meditation, deep breathing, yoga, reading, art, or music.

5. Focus on getting better-quality sleep. Go to bed earlier; keep your room dark and cool.

But here's the really cool part: Your neuromuscular system adapts to strength training superfast. In the first month of your 90-day program, your strength will improve so quickly that you'll probably need to choose heavier weights for a few exercises to get a good workout.

Weeks 4 to 6: You May Look Bigger—But You're Not

It is physiologically impossible for hypertrophy to occur in the first 4 to 6 weeks of strength training. So why do your muscles look bigger in the mirror?

Any new activity causes some degree of stress in your body. Even at low intensity levels, this stress causes water redistribution throughout the tissues of your body. Strength training in particular causes just a bit more shake-up. In the first few weeks of your workouts, you are going to experience water retention. It may look like muscle growth, but it's actually just a swelling of sorts. Even if your initial workouts aren't very challenging, you will experience this water redistribution. If your workouts *are* challenging, more water rushes in to your muscles to help them recover. This means a bit more water retention or swelling.

So don't worry that you are bulking up during the first few weeks of strength training. Water swelling up your muscles is common. The best thing you can do is stay consistent in your workouts, foster good recovery, and stay strong under pressure. After this initial phase, your body will adapt and release and recirculate any water it has retained.

After Week 6: Patience Pays Off

Around the 6-week mark, true hypertrophy begins to occur if you are giving your muscles sufficient time under tension. This is where the good stuff starts to happen! Your muscles begin to grow and become more influential on your metabolism and your ability to get lean. Exciting!

Some women might experience a phase where the muscle begins to grow and pushes body fat outward. Some mistake this phase as bulk, when in reality it is simply a short-lived phase before a substantial decrease in body fat. Lean muscle mass is instrumental in decreasing your body fat, but it is not a direct process. Lean muscle mass helps to boost your metabolism and improve a variety of body functions and that eventually improves your ability to burn off excess body fat.

During this second phase, if you start to feel bulky before your body fat decreases, hold tight and stay consistent with your workouts. This is a short-lived phase before your body comes full circle in changing its composition. Stick with your plan.

Research shows that strength training can significantly decrease your body fat and increase your lean muscle by 12 weeks. Consider a study from McMaster University in Canada where young women did heavy strength training 5 days a week for 12 weeks. They also supplemented their training with milk (a good source of protein and carbs). The subjects gained 4 pounds of muscle and lost 3.5 pounds of fat! Remember, muscle is more dense than fat, so their body size actually decreased.

In another study, researchers from Brazil recruited 20 elderly women for a strength-training program where they increased the load each week. The women trained three times per week for 16 weeks. Can you guess what happened at the end of the study? That's right, they gained muscle and lost fat. Specifically, they added 5 pounds of muscle and lost more than 16 pounds of fat.

That's worth repeating: In three strength workouts a week over the course of 16 weeks, women lost 16 pounds of fat and gained 5 pounds of muscle! Ahhh-mazing! And if you are younger than those women, you can expect even better results.

Still Worried about Bulk?

You will increase the size of your muscles using the 90-day programs. But don't worry—you will not look like a bro. Without the help of anabolic steroids, you are absolutely unable to develop muscle like a man. Muscle growth is heavily dependent on testosterone, and you have one-tenth the amount of a man. You literally do not have the hormonal profile to be able to build big, scary muscles. Instead, you have an ability to develop your musculature. You'll build long, firm, sexy muscle that will make your body shed fat and stay lean for life, as long as you:

> Stay committed and consistent with your training.

> Eat a healthy diet that fuels your workouts properly.

> Consistently challenge your muscles by pushing them beyond their current capabilities (the Last 2 Reps Rule in the next chapter will make that really easy to do).

Chapter 6
The Three-Step System to Strength

Very rarely do I hear women talk about their success when they try strength training. They either complain about lackluster results or about being discouraged by soreness and fatigue from the workouts. No wonder there are so few women in the weights section at the gym!

The main reason why women (and plenty of men, too!) have a poor experience when they lift is because the nuances of strength training can be sooo confusing, and they go at it without a plan in place. To gain all those terrific health benefits in Chapter 4 quickly and efficiently, you have to do more than simply pick up a pair of dumbbells and crank out 12 reps. That's like sailing a boat without a rudder. You're moving, but you don't know where you're going, and you couldn't get there anyway because you can't steer. Don't lift weights rudderless. Doing so will often lead to frustration and, worse, injury.

You need an easy-to-remember plan that will keep you on track and help you avoid the mistakes that will cause unnecessary soreness and fatigue—and really bum you out. My three-step system will guarantee that you lift right, and it will give you confidence by automatically answering common questions like:

"How much weight should I use?" and *"Am I working hard enough?"*

So what are the three steps? Simple.

1. Technique
2. Speed of Movement
3. The Last 2 Reps Rule

Let's dig into each one.

1. Technique

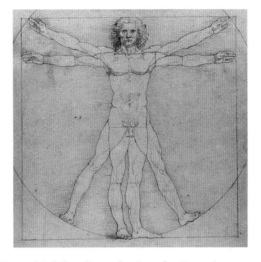

They say technique trumps all, and it's so true in the gym. Why? Because proper lifting technique is what will ultimately give you beautiful, symmetrical, sexy body proportions. Poor technique often creates muscle imbalances that aren't very attractive and can cause pain and injury.

You've seen the image at right before, haven't you?

It's Leonardo da Vinci's *Vitruvian Man*, which he drew during the Renaissance, around 1490. It is sometimes referred to as the *Canon of Proportions* because it depicts the ideal human proportions from a geometrical perspective. Da Vinci was inspired to create this image by an ancient Roman architect, Vitruvius, who established that the ideal human body demonstrates very specific proportions. The text below the drawing (text not shown here) reads, "From the roots of the hair to the bottom of the chin is the tenth of a man's height; from the bottom of the chin to the top of his head is one eighth of his height; from the top of the breast to the top of his head will be one sixth of a man . . . " and so on.

This image establishes the human body as an expression of art, geometry, architecture, and nature all in one. Da Vinci saw the workings of the human body as an analogy for the workings of the universe.

That gives me chills! One of the world's most prolific visionaries is showing us through the human body that science and nature are linked. Our bodies are brilliantly designed, and that tells me that we are here for a purpose. The body is not just a vehicle to get you through the day.

Beauty and Function

Symmetry and proportion appeal to the human eye. It is why a flower or a landscape can stop you in your tracks and a beautiful person makes you stare. When you see a beautiful body, you don't realize it but you are responding to notes of mathematics, art, nature, and science.

Balance and proportion are also critical to function. The phrase "form follows function" in architecture means that a physical structure, such as a building, should represent its intended function. Your body follows the same laws. Every single muscle in your body has a very precise role. Each muscle is designed to resist gravity in order to keep you aligned throughout every movement you make. Therefore, some muscles are bigger and stronger because they do most of the work. Other muscles are more like support beams that assist the overall integrity of the structure.

Your foundation is your lower body—the muscles of your legs, which support and align your pelvis, spine, shoulders, and neck. Just like a building, this foundation needs to be level, balanced, and strong in all the right places to keep the upper structures in optimal alignment. This is the main reason why the muscles below your waist are the biggest in your body. Your legs carry your entire body weight, constantly adjusting to keep you balanced as you move. Your leg muscles work in conjunction with your glutes (butt muscles) for all locomotion.

When muscles are out of proportion and symmetry—say, one side of your body is stronger or more developed than the other—your structural alignment is off. Even a slight misalignment can cause wear and tear on a specific joint or muscle, triggering soreness and pain. In fact, it's not accidents and injuries that cause most chronic aches and pains, it's muscle imbalance, poor posture, and weak supporting muscles. And where there's strain, there's also drain. Poor body proportion and alignment drain your energy, making you feel tired even after a good night's rest. Remember: Strong muscles equal strong energy.

The most common muscular weaknesses I see in women are in the

> Hip stabilizers (the muscles in your hips that keep you aligned as you walk or run)
> Glutes (butt muscles)
> Hamstrings (the muscles on the back of your thighs)
> Core (abs and lower back)
> Shoulder stabilizers (the muscles that keep your shoulders in proper alignment)

Women are more susceptible than men to muscular imbalance because of the way the pelvis is structured. You are blessed with wider hips for childbirth. But this creates more extreme angles in your lower body, which means some muscles work harder than others, causing imbalance and poor alignment. The muscles on the front of your thigh (your quadriceps) should be stronger than the muscles on the back of your thigh (your hamstrings) by about 25 percent. If this ratio is off, it may affect the mechanics of the knee and hip joints, causing undue stress on the tendons and ligaments, including the ACL (anterior cruciate ligament), which is particularly troublesome and common for women. But proper exercise selection and performance technique can fix these imbalances. I've taken care of the exercise picks; all four 90-day training programs feature exercises chosen to address common female body alignment problems. Your job will be to master each exercise by practicing proper technique, using the step-by-step photos and exercise descriptions with key performance pointers in Chapter 7.

Are You Using Too Much Weight?

A common mistake is to assume that strength-training workouts should be hard and heavy. It's a *strength*-training workout after all, right? Yes, but the

Choosing the Right Weight for You

When you are first getting acquainted with the equipment in your gym, figuring out ideal weight loads to begin with takes some trial and error. Here are some ballpark starting weight loads that you can use as a very general guideline for your first workout.

Suggested Starting Weight Loads

Leg Press—50 to 70 pounds

Walking Lunge—0 (body weight only) to 10 pounds

Leg Extension—20 to 50 pounds

Reverse Grip Pulldown—30 to 50 pounds

Seated Upright Chest Fly—20 to 40 pounds

Barbell Overhead Press—20 to 30 pounds

Dumbbell Bent Arm Side Raise—5 to 8 pounds

Dumbbell Hammer Curl—5 to 10 pounds

Dumbbell French Press—5 to 8 pounds

Calf Raise—20 to 30 pounds

At the beginning of your first workout, pick a starting weight and assess how it feels at around the 5th or 6th repetition. Does it feel superhard, supereasy, or just right? If it's either extreme, stop the set, adjust the weight appropriately, rest for 1 minute, and begin again.

goal is to identify your current strength level in all muscle groups and then expose them to weight loads that are just a bit harder. The goal isn't to lift as heavy as possible and sacrifice technique. You want to fatigue your muscle, but only to the point where it can still manage the movement with excellent technique.

For that reason, minding your technique is an easy way to ensure that you are using the proper amount of weight. If you find your technique is suffering, you could be trying to "cheat the weight up" in order to complete a repetition with a weight that is too heavy. That alone can cause muscular imbalance and injury.

Let's turn our backs toward the problem to illustrate what happens when your technique isn't right.

Consider two important back muscles: your latissimus dorsi (or lats) and trapezius (or traps). Your lats, which cover your shoulder blades, are very important. Their job is to bring your arms toward your body in a pulling motion and keep your shoulder joints in an optimal place during movement and at rest. The lats are chronically underutilized and often the source for muscular imbalance.

Just above your lats toward your neck are your traps, which run from your head down and out toward your shoulders and then down the middle of your back. These guys are responsible for pulling your entire shoulder joints up toward your ears—the movement you make with your shoulders when you are cold and shiver—and a prime source of neck and shoulder tension, muscle "knots," and even shoulder joint injuries. We humans hold a lot of stress in our traps, so they tend to get overused and become dominant back muscles. Look in the mirror the next time you're feeling stressed. Are you holding your shoulders up by your ears? Not so attractive, is it? Big thick traps aren't either. From an aesthetic perspective, you look more elegant and feminine when your shoulders are released down, slightly drawn back, and your neck muscles are relaxed.

It is important to exercise your lats to strengthen and balance them against the dominant traps. The Reverse Grip Pulldown exercise (see page 44) is perfect for doing just that. But it will only work if you use the proper amount of weight and the proper technique. If your weight load is too heavy, your domineering traps will kick into gear and do the work, ignoring your lats.

Mirror, Mirror

There's a reason why the gym walls are covered with mirrors, besides making it easier for guys to admire their biceps and adjust their hair. Mirrors reflect your lifting technique right back at you. Use them to check your form and fix it if it's not right.

Key Points: *Technique*

Technique is the most important consideration during your workouts for three reasons.

1. It forces weaker muscles to step up.
2. It allows dominant muscles to settle down.
3. It creates a visually beautiful work of art.

Repeat after me: "Technique trumps all!"

So incorrect form means that your lats won't get the attention they need to become stronger and that the traps will continue to dominate. This is why technique is so important, and only the proper weight for your muscles' ability will allow you to perform an exercise with flawless technique. If you make technique your first priority and execute every set following all three steps, you'll know without a doubt that you're using the proper weight. Just starting out? See "Choosing the Right Weight for You" on page 42 for a good general guide.

How you *perform* the exercises during your workouts is the most critical factor in an *effective* resistance program.

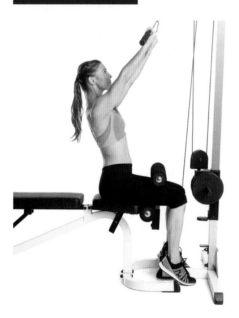
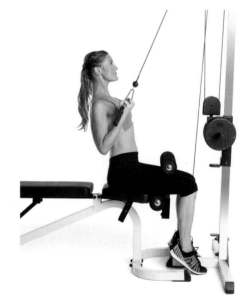

Proper technique for the Reverse Grip Pulldown.

2. Speed of Movement

Speed of movement—the tempo at which you raise and lower a weight—is often ignored by lifters, even by pro trainers and athletes. Yet it might be the most important variable for developing strength. It's a real game changer, and that's why it's the second step in this system.

What's "Time under Tension"?

The amount of time the muscle spends under exertion. There is a correlation between time under tension and strength development. More time under tension = more strength.

Every exercise included in the 90-day training programs at the back of this book features two movement phases: the effort phase (labeled "HARD" in the exercise instructions) and the release phase (marked "EASY"). The effort, or Hard, phase is where you put the "work" into "workout." It is the phase of movement where you have to exert yourself by pushing or pulling with your arms or legs primarily. The release, or Easy, phase is typically when you lower the weight or release its tension on your body.

Let's use one of my favorite exercises, the Dumbbell Hammer Curl, as an example.

The Dumbbell Hammer Curl

The motion of curling the weights from your thighs to your shoulders by bending your arms is the Hard phase. Straightening your arms to lower the weight back to your thighs is the Easy phase.

The technical name for the Hard movement phase is concentric contraction. All it really means is that the muscle shortens to create movement. When you lift the weight in the Dumbbell Hammer Curl, for example, your biceps shorten to make your arm move.

What's special about this phase is that it responds very well to powerful and forceful effort. You will get more out of your strength-training workouts if you exaggerate this movement with force. Some of my colleagues call this performing an "explosive" movement. But I think that encourages too much speed. If you explode too much during your sets, you run a great risk of injury. I prefer to think in terms of being "enthusiastic on the Hard." Practically speaking, I'd like you to take 2 seconds to complete this phase of the lift. That's pretty quick and forceful but not overdoing it. In the example of the biceps curl, you would raise the weight to your shoulder to a two-count.

The technical name for the Easy movement phase is eccentric contraction. It means that the muscle is lengthening to produce the movement. This phase is when your muscle actually develops strength. How cool is that? The Easy phase is actually more important than the Hard phase!

It is during this lengthening contraction—typically when you lower the weight back to the starting position—that muscle has a great propensity to become stronger. Therefore, you want to emphasize this phase. Remember back

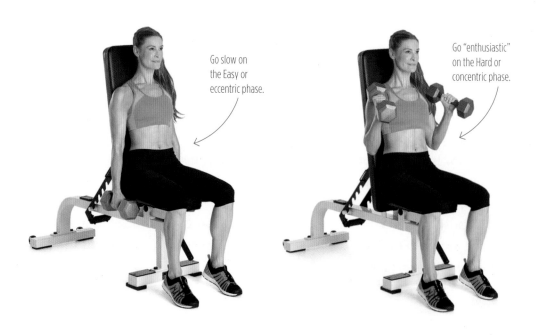

Go slow on the Easy or eccentric phase.

Go "enthusiastic" on the Hard or concentric phase.

when I talked about time under tension? The Easy phase is when you expose your muscles to more time under tension. That's why I say, "Slow on the Easy." You should take a full 4 seconds to gradually release the weight back to the starting position. In the example of the biceps curl, you'll lower the weight back to your thighs to a four-count. If it helps, count "one Mississippi . . . two Mississippi . . ." and so on. And remember your technique while performing both the Hard and Easy phases: No rocking to use momentum! Rocking and using momentum are particularly common in the biceps curl.

Key Points:
Speed of Movement

1. Enthusiastic on the Hard (2 seconds)
2. Pause at the hardest point (2 seconds)
3. Slow on the Easy (4 seconds)

As you perform the Easy phase, concentrate on using the active muscle or muscle group in a very deliberate way to get the most benefit and ensure muscle contraction. Visualize controlling the active muscle in a slow manner using perfect technique as you move through the phase. This phase is extra special because it's the key to building strength without adding much size.

The Pause

In between the Hard and Easy phases, there is a moment of transition where the movement reverses. This is called the peak contraction point, and it's also critical to building strength. At this position, you're putting the greatest amount of tension on the muscle without actual movement, which is why it's also known as the isometric contraction point. When you reach this point, I'd like you to pause for 2 seconds. During this isometric two-count, tense your muscles—really squeeze them—to add even more stress, which will ultimately create greater damage to the muscle fibers.

So to review the second step, it's the Hard phase for 2 seconds, pause and squeeze for 2 seconds, the Easy phase for 4 seconds, and then repeat. Note that some exercises begin with the Easy phase and end with the Hard. The Flat Bench Press is a good example. Just remember how to perform Easy and Hard no matter which order they occur in an exercise. You can see how this step can influence the first: technique. If your speed is too fast in either direction, your technique suffers.

Practice your tempo and think, "Enthusiastic on the Hard, pause in between, and slow on the Easy."

Tempo **is the most overlooked** *important* **variable for developing strength.**

3. The Last 2 Reps Rule

As you learned in Chapter 5, the only way your muscles can grow stronger is if you force them to perform beyond their current abilities. You must challenge them with progressive resistance. Even if you performed an exercise with perfect technique, using proper speed of movement, you wouldn't gain strength and muscle tone if you didn't expose your muscles to the stimulus created by overload.

Enter Step 3: the Last 2 Reps Rule. This means that you should use enough weight so that the last 2 repetitions of a set—say, reps 11 and 12 of a 12-rep set—are very difficult to perform. The weight used should be light enough to perform the set with awesome technique and proper tempo—**except for the last 2 reps.** That's when fatigue sets in and your excellent technique begins to break down. But it's also when you tax your muscles to the max, causing real change. The stress of those last 2 reps under tension causes extra muscle microtears that lead to strength and muscle gains in recovery.

So what do those last 2 tough reps look like? Well, if I were standing next to you, I would want to see a bit of a struggle going on, with about 70 or 80 percent of perfect form. All other reps during a given set should feel really good, strong, and effective. Then, as you approach the last 2 reps, you should have to say to yourself, "Okay, this is work." You should have to step up, dig in, and be strong. In my opinion, this is where the workout begins. The last 2 reps are the most important of every set. This is where you create real change in your body.

When You Just . . . Can't . . . Lift . . . It . . . Again

As you gain confidence, you may be able to attempt weight loads where your technique is great for all of the reps leading up to the last 2, and then you stall out completely. Hooray! This is called momentary muscle failure (MMF), and it's where the good stress occurs that demands the activation of new muscle fibers, triggering muscle growth. MMF won't occur every set, and it often happens only once or twice during a workout.

When MMF happens, continue pushing or pulling during the reps that seem to be stalling out. There will be a moment when you realize that you are unable to finish the last 2 reps and your movement will literally stop in the middle of the Hard phase. The first few times it happens, you will most likely realize the "failure" is coming, and you will instantaneously give up. Once again, this is your body's cunning survival instinct keeping you safe from the big, scary, "dangerous" threat! But get comfortable leaning in to this moment. Be brave and allow your muscles to continue pushing or pulling for a beat or two even though movement has stalled out. Huge progress occurs in this split second when your brain says, "Keep working!" even though you are stalling out. A strong electrical signal gets sent from your brain to the working muscles telling them to step up, which recruits new muscle fibers. You must fail to succeed. And remember: This is a reason you should work out with a partner to spot you whenever you lift weight over your chest or head. Momentary muscle failure shouldn't result in broken bones! Be safe!

There will be a moment during these reps when your survival instinct kicks in and your mind tells you that you can't do it. For a split second, you'll want to give up. You will feel an emotion, possibly anger or fear, that tells you it's not worth it. That is your moment to redefine yourself. Dig for that deep strength that lives inside of you. You are so much stronger than you think. The last 2 reps of a hard set are where your "failures" end and your strength begins. Embrace the discomfort. In the end, it's only a moment in time. This moment holds the key to changing your life in ways that you can only imagine. If you can embrace the discomfort and fight your doubts, you will harness massive ability for

Know Your Equipment

There are a few things you should know about the equipment that you'll be using. Dumbbells and machines are pretty self-explanatory, but here are some important details for barbells.

Barbells come in many sizes. Most likely your gym will have a standard Olympic bar in place for the Flat Bench Press. This bar weighs 45 pounds. While you can use this same bar for other exercises, I recommend seeking out shorter barbells (weighing 25 to 35 pounds) for the following movements:

Bent-Over Barbell Row
Deadlift
Barbell Overhead Press

For these exercises, you can use the bar alone for your workouts. At some point, you will most likely want to begin adding weight to the bar. Weight plates range from 2.5 to 45 pounds. When you're ready to add plates to your bar, always use the metal clips to secure the weight plates. **Insider tip:** The metal clips aren't just to keep the weights from sliding off the bar. More importantly, they keep the weight plates from shifting during your set. Even small shifts cause the bar to become imbalanced, which means that one side of your body will end up compensating to account for the weight difference. It might be a small detail, but this kind of thing promotes body imbalances and asymmetry. Always use the clips to make sure your bod is bangin' from every angle!

change. You will also discover an incredible sense of accomplishment.

As you enter the uncomfortable phase—the most important last 2 reps of the set—I want you to say to yourself: "Just try."

Just try to complete the set and work through the last 2 reps. Instead of shying away from the challenge, lean into it and embrace it. Face the discomfort and see what happens. Breathe. You can do it, and it will be worth the effort.

You are *so* much *stronger* than you think.

Key Points: *The Last 2 Reps Rule*

1. The last 2 reps are crucial to creating real change in your body.

2. Your chosen weight should be heavy enough so that you struggle and really need to push yourself.

3. You are using heavy enough weight and doing this right if you perform the last 2 reps at about 70 to 80 percent of perfect form.

Chapter 7
Strength Exercises for the Feminine Body

You didn't learn how to ice-skate or braid hair or even fry an egg without a little trial and error. Anything that requires some skill takes good instruction (with illustrations) and some practice. So don't feel intimidated by strength-training exercises. First, you learn how to perform the move and understand what it does for your body, and then you practice your technique in the gym until you get it down. Everybody started the same way. Even I stumbled a few times until I got it. You'll pick it up quickly.

For *The 12-Week Head-to-Toe Transformation,* I've selected the best strength- and muscle-building exercises for women at any level of fitness. The movements are organized by muscle groups, beginning with lower-body exercises, and include performance pointers that highlight the key tips for perfect form. The main thing to remember is to breathe naturally (don't hold your breath, which is a common beginner's mistake) while doing these exercises. Your brain and body don't function well without oxygen! And keep in mind the Three-Step System to Strength you learned in the previous chapter.

I tried to make these instructions as easy as possible; for example, you'll

Let's Go to the Video

Want to watch a video demonstration of an exercise?

Visit womenshealthmag.com and my new Web site, womensstrengthnation.com, to find instructional videos, post questions, and share your success story.

see the words HARD and EASY corresponding to the two different phases of movement reviewed in Chapter 6. Remember, HARD identifies the part of the move that requires the most enthusiastic effort, such as the pressing portion of the Leg Press, when you extend your legs out straight. You'll recall that you are to take 2 seconds to complete this phase of the lift. EASY refers to the part of the exercise where you release the weight, such as when you lower dumbbells in a Biceps Curl. You will take 4 seconds to gradually release the weight back to the starting position. Move quickly on HARD and slowly on EASY. And pause briefly during the transition. Starting on the next page, you'll find the exercises for all four Lift to Get Lean workout programs.

LEG PRESS

STRENGTHENS

QUADRICEPS, HAMSTRINGS, GLUTES

STARTING POSITION

Begin with your feet on the upper portion of the footplate with your toes turned open to about 11:00 and 1:00 (see inset). Extend your legs to press the weight up and keep your knees unlocked. Allow a natural arch in your lower back and anchor down with your hands **(A)**.

MOVEMENT

Slowly lower the footplate toward you by bending your knees and allow your knees to track toward your shoulders **(B)**. **EASY**

Pause with your knees at or below 90 degrees.

Then push into your heels and return to the starting position **(A)** without locking your knees. **HARD**

Why It's Perfect for You

I love this exercise because it is custom-made for the female body and it targets the hamstrings and glutes, which are often weak in women. Because you are seated and fully supported, it is ultra safe and allows you to direct all of your concentration and power to your lower body.

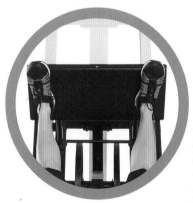

Your feet should be hip-width apart. Turn your toes outward. Because women have wider, more-open hips than men do, this foot position unlocks the alignment of your legs, allowing you to better activate the muscles of the lower body.

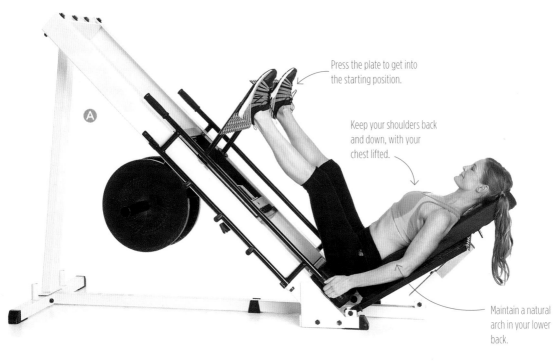

Ⓐ

Press the plate to get into
the starting position.

Keep your shoulders back
and down, with your
chest lifted.

Maintain a natural
arch in your lower
back.

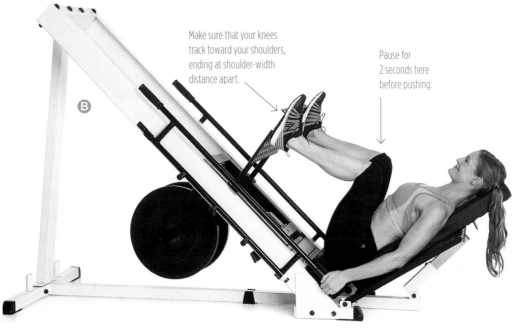

Ⓑ

Make sure that your knees
track toward your shoulders,
ending at shoulder-width
distance apart.

Pause for
2 seconds here
before pushing.

LEG CURL

STRENGTHENS

HAMSTRINGS

STARTING POSITION

Position yourself so that your knees are just below the pad of the weight machine and the padded ankle roller hits between your calf muscle and your Achilles tendon.

With feet flexed, turn them out to 11:00 and 1:00. Slightly arch your lower back. Grab the handles **(A)**.

ADVANCED ALTERNATIVE

Position yourself as described above, but rise up on your elbows, keeping them just under your shoulders (see inset). This option isolates the hamstrings even more and is therefore more challenging.

MOVEMENT

Keeping your feet flexed, contract your hamstrings and pull your heels toward your butt **(B)**. **HARD**

Pause without changing the arch in your lower back.

Then slowly lower your heels back to the start **(A)**. **EASY**

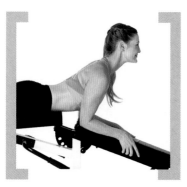

Keep your chest lifted up and outward if performing the Advanced version.

Why It's Perfect for You

Strengthening and toning the hamstrings will make the backs of your thighs look awesome. This move concentrates the resistance completely on this often weak muscle group as the knee flexes. What's more, the exercise strengthens the muscles and tendons surrounding the knee joint, which is important for women, especially since they are particularly prone to knee injuries like ACL tears.

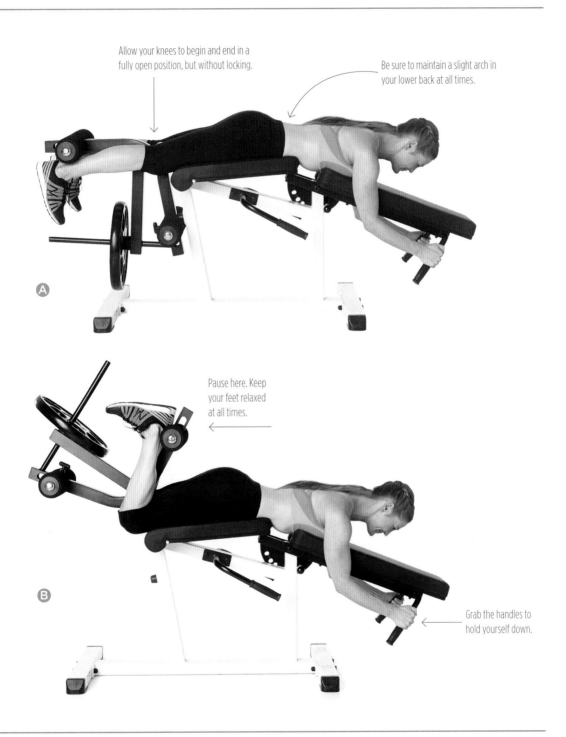

Allow your knees to begin and end in a fully open position, but without locking.

Be sure to maintain a slight arch in your lower back at all times.

A

Pause here. Keep your feet relaxed at all times.

B

Grab the handles to hold yourself down.

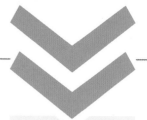

WALKING LUNGE

STRENGTHENS

HAMSTRINGS, GLUTES, QUADRICEPS

STARTING POSITION

Stand with your feet together and your arms at your sides holding dumbbells. Stand tall with your shoulders back and down, and keep your knees unlocked.

MOVEMENT

Take a large step forward with your right leg, landing on your right heel with your toes turned out to 1:00 **(A)**. Allow your back leg to relax so that your knee drops toward the floor. **EASY**

Pause briefly here with your weight on your right heel.

Push into your right heel to stand up and step forward, returning to the starting position **(B)**. **HARD** Immediately step forward onto your left leg and repeat the movement **(C)**, alternating sides as you move forward in space.

Why It's Perfect for You

Because you are moving forward in space, this exercise mimics the natural movements of walking and running, strengthening the related muscles. It puts the ideal amount of good stress on your hamstrings and glutes.

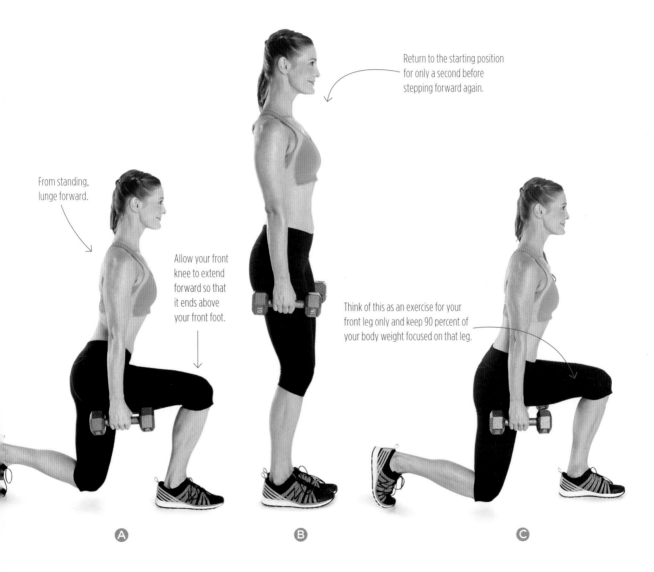

From standing,
lunge forward.

Allow your front
knee to extend
forward so that
it ends above
your front foot.

Return to the starting position
for only a second before
stepping forward again.

Think of this as an exercise for your
front leg only and keep 90 percent of
your body weight focused on that leg.

(A)

(B)

(C)

LEG EXTENSION

STRENGTHENS

QUADRICEPS, TIBIALIS ANTERIOR (FRONT OF SHIN)

STARTING POSITION

Adjust the seat and ankle arm so you are positioned with your knees next to the rotation joint of the leg extension machine and the ankle arm is just above your feet. Allow a natural arch in your lower back. Anchor yourself by holding the handles of the machine. Flex your feet with your toes turned outward at 11:00 and 1:00 **(A)**.

MOVEMENT

Contract your thighs and extend your legs outward until your knees are fully open, nearing a locked position **(B)**. **HARD**

Pause with your legs fully extended and straight, feet flexed toward you.

Slowly bend your knees and lower your feet back to the starting position under control **(A)**. **EASY**

Be conservative and use lighter weights to start.

Why It's Perfect for You

The female body's wide hips, while custom-made for childbearing, cause a pronounced weakness of the quadriceps. This exercise corrects any imbalances among the four quadriceps muscles to promote healthy knee alignment and tracking.

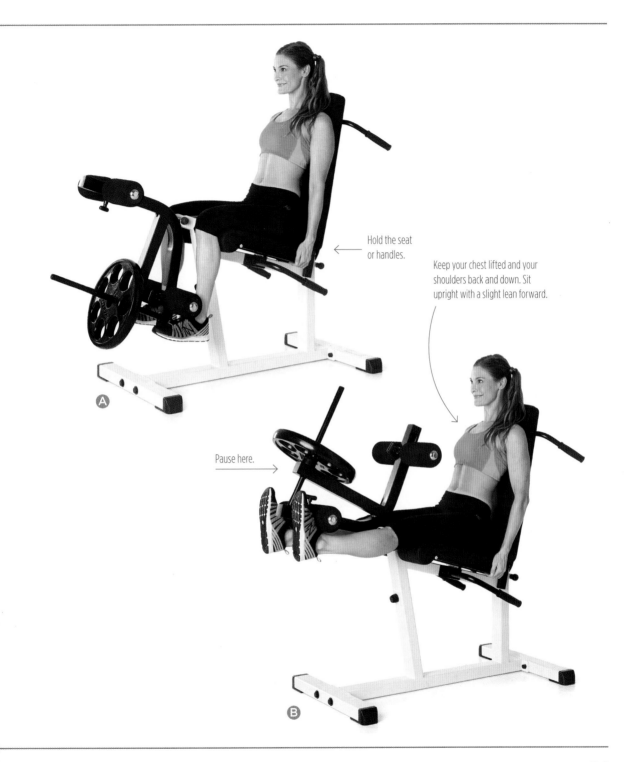

Hold the seat
or handles.

Keep your chest lifted and your
shoulders back and down. Sit
upright with a slight lean forward.

A

Pause here.

B

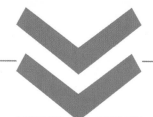

GOBLET SQUAT

STRENGTHENS

GLUTES, HAMSTRINGS, QUADRICEPS, CORE

STARTING POSITION

Stand with your feet shoulder-width apart and toes pointing to 10:00 and 2:00. Hold one end of a dumbbell against your chest, keeping contact throughout the movement **(A)**. Stand tall with your knees unlocked.

MOVEMENT

Allow your hips to drop straight down, ending with your butt below your knees and your chest lifted **(B)**. **EASY**

Pause at the bottom, but keep tension on your heels and butt.

Press into your heels, keep your posture tall, and lift straight up as you return to the starting position **(A)**. **HARD**

Why It's Perfect for You

This version of a traditional squat puts your hips in an unlocked position so that you can activate all of the related muscles better. Other squat variations tend to emphasize the quadriceps. This version puts more emphasis on the glutes, hamstrings, and core stabilizing muscles. It is hands down my favorite squat for women.

Keep your abs engaged (see inset 1) and maintain a slight arch in your lower back (see inset 2).

Visualize how a baby plops down into a squat position from standing and try to mimic the movement. Simply let your hips drop down in a relaxed manner while keeping your chest lifted high and your back straight.

Extras: You may be wondering: Why not do a Back Squat or a Barbell Hack Squat? Well, those traditional squats work great for men because of their narrow and closed pelvis. For women, these versions restrict movement in the knees and hips and put more emphasis on the quadriceps. Women are already quad dominant and need to balance this with more posterior chain exercises like this one. This version emphasizes the glutes and hamstrings.

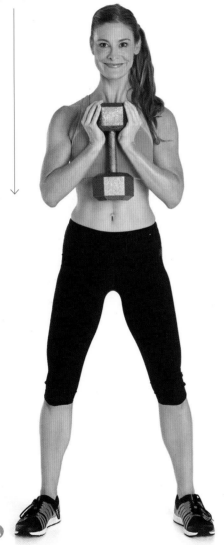

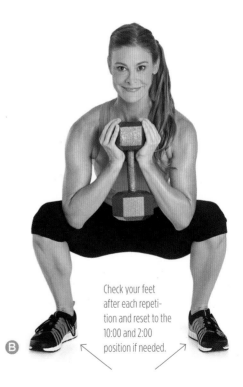

Check your feet after each repetition and reset to the 10:00 and 2:00 position if needed.

BENCH STEPUP

STRENGTHENS

GLUTES, HAMSTRINGS, QUADRICEPS, CORE

STARTING POSITION

Stand facing a stable bench or step, holding dumbbells at your sides. Place your right foot onto the bench with your toes turned out to 1:00, and lean slightly forward. Keep a slight arch in your lower back throughout the exercise **(A)**.

MOVEMENT

Press into the arch of your right foot and step onto the bench. **HARD**

Bring your left foot up to stabilize your balance **(B)**, then immediately step back down with your left foot, ending in the starting position **(A)** and leaving your right foot on the bench. **EASY**

Keeping tension on your right leg at the starting position, pause before pressing back up onto the bench with your right leg. You will repeat all reps on the right leg before switching feet.

Why It's Perfect for You

This movement is called a "level change," meaning you raise or lower your entire body, and is important for optimal lower-body function. This kind of movement keeps you strong for climbing stairs and other everyday activities. It's also a cool exercise because technically it focuses on one leg at a time, but in a way that mimics everyday movement. It emphasizes your hamstrings as hip extensors, bringing balance to your lower-body mechanics.

Extras: The Walking Lunge and Bench Stepup are single-leg exercises that mimic natural human activity, whereas other isolated single-leg exercises may require too much balance for beginners. Focus all of your effort and attention on the movement, not on balance and coordination.

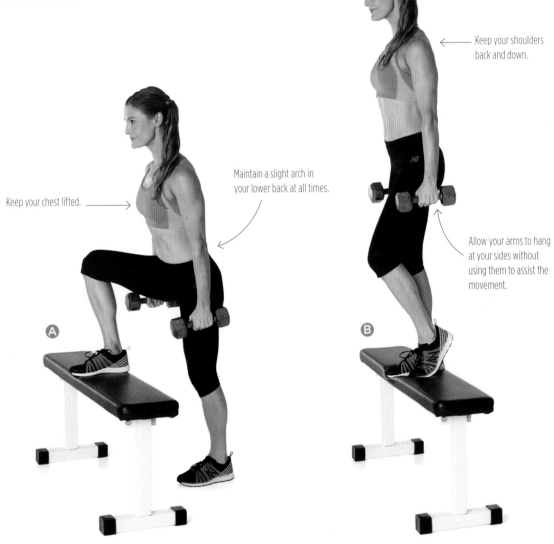

Keep your shoulders back and down.

Keep your chest lifted.

Maintain a slight arch in your lower back at all times.

Allow your arms to hang at your sides without using them to assist the movement.

A

B

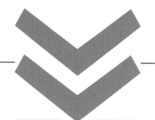

DEADLIFT

Why It's Perfect for You

STRENGTHENS

NEARLY EVERY MUSCLE IN THE BODY. AND THAT'S WHY I LOVE IT.

STARTING POSITION

Begin standing with a shorter barbell in an overhand position in front of your thighs, with hands slightly wider than your shoulders. Keep your chest lifted and your shoulders pulled back and down **(A)**. Turn your feet outward to 11:00 and 1:00 and keep your knees unlocked (see inset). Throughout the exercise, maintain an arch in your lower back and contract your abs.

MOVEMENT

Keep your chest lifted high and bend your knees, allowing your hips to reach back as if sitting into a chair. Keep your arms in a dead hang, and allow the bar to slide down your legs **(B)**. **EASY**

Pause at the bottom with the weight plates hovering just above the ground, your hips reaching back and your chest lifted up high.

Keeping your chest lifted, push into your heels, maintain a dead hang with your arms, and push up to the starting position **(A)**. **HARD**

The Deadlift is one of the most revered and important exercises of all. When done properly, it strengthens the entire body in a highly functional way. It is a form of a squat, but because the weight is in front of your body, it works better for women than other squats. In this case, your "pulling" muscles hold the bar, whereas in a traditional squat, your "pushing" muscles hold the weight. Women are built for pulling, not pushing.

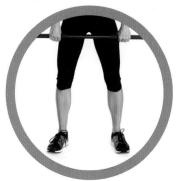

Your feet should be shoulder-width apart and toes turned outward slightly.

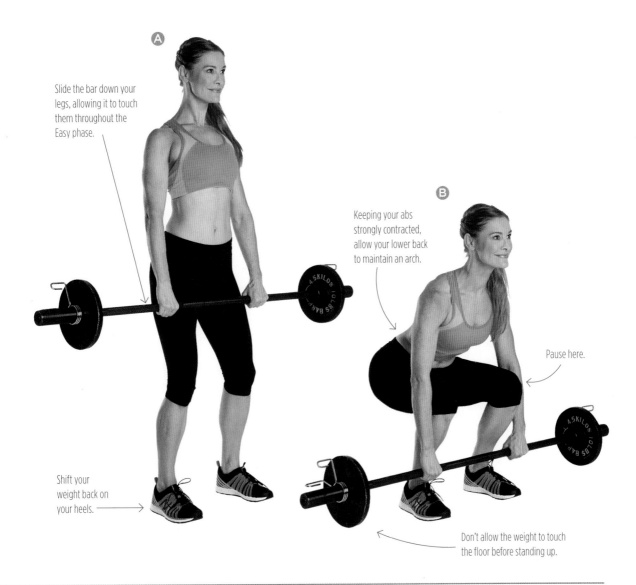

A

Slide the bar down your legs, allowing it to touch them throughout the Easy phase.

Shift your weight back on your heels.

B

Keeping your abs strongly contracted, allow your lower back to maintain an arch.

Pause here.

Don't allow the weight to touch the floor before standing up.

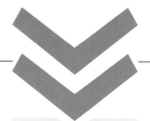

CALF RAISE

STRENGTHENS

CALVES, LOWER LEG STABILIZERS

STARTING POSITION

Stand on a stable box or stair step so that half of each foot is off the box or stair and your body weight is on the balls of your feet. Your feet should be parallel to the floor. Hold a dumbbell in the vertical position tightly to your chest. Stand tall and allow a natural curve in your lower back **(A)**.

MOVEMENT

Mentally focus your attention on your core for balance, and slowly rise up onto your toes **(B)**. **HARD**

Pause at the top and squeeze your calves to rise as high as possible.

Slowly lower back down until your heels are just a tiny bit below parallel to the floor. **EASY**

Why It's Perfect for You

Calf Raises improve ankle and lower leg function, helping to support all of your activities. Improved balance and stability in your ankles and feet are essential for injury prevention. Ankles are often neglected, and strong ankles and lower legs are the foundation of everything that you do. This movement appears in all of my 90-day training programs because it is so important. Make time to perform it!

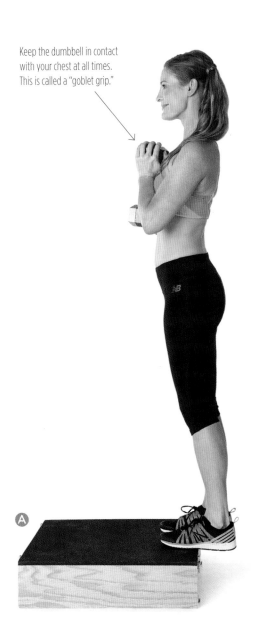

Keep the dumbbell in contact
with your chest at all times.
This is called a "goblet grip."

A

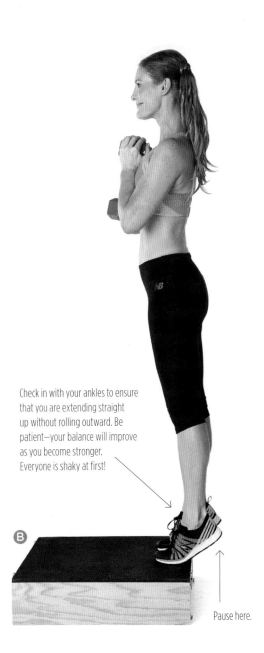

Check in with your ankles to ensure
that you are extending straight
up without rolling outward. Be
patient—your balance will improve
as you become stronger.
Everyone is shaky at first!

B

Pause here.

REVERSE GRIP PULLDOWN

STRENGTHENS

LATS (BACK), BICEPS, SHOULDERS

STARTING POSITION

Sit with your knees securely anchored under the lat machine's pad. Raise your arms and grasp the bar hanging from the cable with your hands shoulder-width apart and palms facing you, which is called an *underhand grip*. Lean back slightly, lift your chest upward, and pull your shoulders back and down. Keep your arms fully extended without locking elbows **(A)**. See inset 1.

MOVEMENT

Bring your shoulder blades together and use your upper back muscles to pull your arms toward you **(B)**. **HARD**

Pause with the bar close to your upper chest, and squeeze your shoulder blades together (see inset 2).

Keeping your shoulders pulled back and down, straighten your arms to allow the bar to return to the starting position **(A)**. **EASY**

Why It's Perfect for You

The reverse-grip hand position puts more emphasis on your back and tightens up the area around your underarm without creating width. This is the best remedy for bra bulge under the arm and around the back, trouble zones for many women. This movement also strengthens and tightens the triceps (the backs of the arms). This is an important exercise for shoulder health and injury prevention.

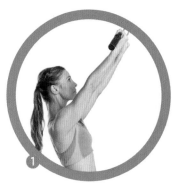

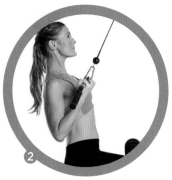

During the pause, allow an arch in your lower back and aggressively contract your upper back.

Extras: I reverse the traditional overhand position on this exercise for two reasons: (1) It is not the ideal positioning for optimal shoulder function. (2) The overhand position causes a widening of the shoulders and upper back. Men like this "cobra look" on themselves. But we women don't care for building these "wings."

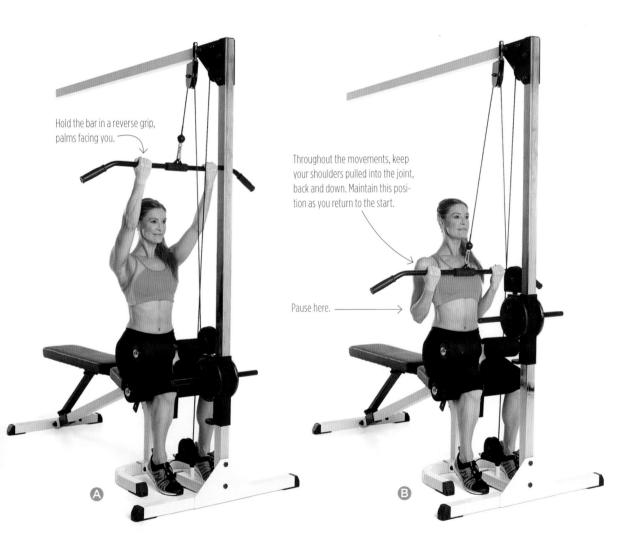

Hold the bar in a reverse grip, palms facing you.

Throughout the movements, keep your shoulders pulled into the joint, back and down. Maintain this position as you return to the start.

Pause here.

A

B

SEATED CABLE ROW

STRENGTHENS

MIDDLE AND UPPER BACK, SHOULDERS

STARTING POSITION

Clip a "double D" handle to the cable and sit down, placing your feet securely on the footplate. Keep your knees bent, maintain a slight arch in your lower back, and lift your chest with your shoulders drawn back. Grasp the handles with each hand, palms facing each other **(A)**.

MOVEMENT

Bring your shoulder blades together as you pull your elbows back and your hands toward your torso **(B)**. **HARD**

Pause with your hands just above your navel, your chest forward and your shoulders drawn back and down.

Keeping your shoulders back and down, allow your arms to extend and return to the starting position **(A)**. **EASY**

Why It's Perfect for You

Similar to the Reverse Grip Pull-down, this movement strengthens your back without creating width between your shoulders. By actively pushing your shoulders down throughout the movement, you get functional core strength as well. It also makes your upper back look awesome!

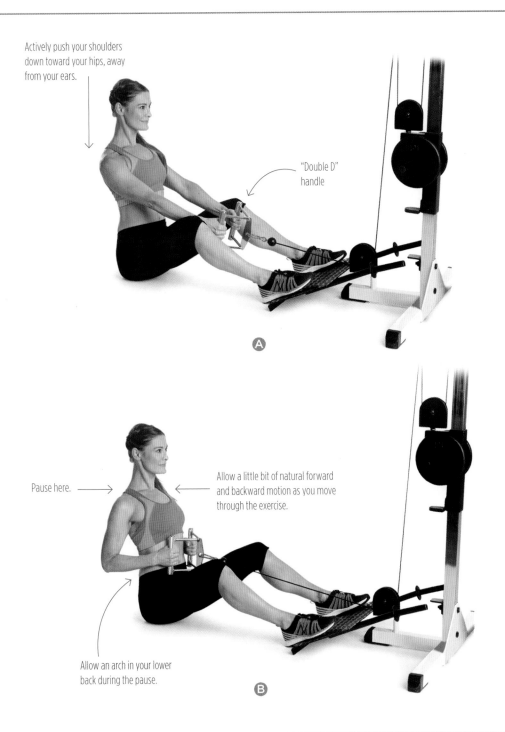

Actively push your shoulders down toward your hips, away from your ears.

"Double D" handle

Ⓐ

Pause here.

Allow a little bit of natural forward and backward motion as you move through the exercise.

Allow an arch in your lower back during the pause.

Ⓑ

BENT-OVER BARBELL ROW

STRENGTHENS

MIDDLE AND UPPER BACK, BICEPS, CORE

STARTING POSITION

Grasp a shorter barbell with your hands shoulder-width apart and palms facing out. Separate your feet by 2 to 4 inches and allow your arms to hang down toward your knees. Bend your knees and reach your hips back until your hands are in front of your knees. Keeping your abs strongly engaged, allow a slight arch in your lower back **(A)**.

MOVEMENT

Bring your shoulder blades together and pull the bar toward you until it touches your torso just above your navel **(B)**. **HARD**

Pause with the bar touching your torso, your chest forward and your shoulders back and down.

Keeping your shoulders drawn inward, release the bar back to the start **(A)**. **EASY**

Why It's Perfect for You

The traditional wide stance will put too much pressure on your lower back because of your wider hips. You'll feel more stable (and protect your lower back) if you keep your feet close together. By bending forward at an angle, this exercise hits the back at the bottom of the shoulder blades to improve shoulder stability. The narrow underhand grip allows you to strengthen your back without creating width. The hand position puts emphasis on the biceps.

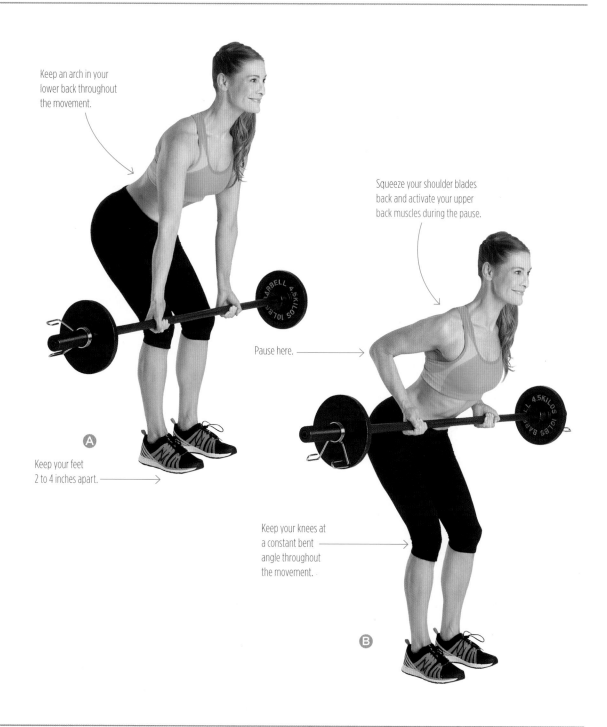

Keep an arch in your lower back throughout the movement.

Squeeze your shoulder blades back and activate your upper back muscles during the pause.

Pause here.

Ⓐ

Keep your feet 2 to 4 inches apart.

Keep your knees at a constant bent angle throughout the movement.

Ⓑ

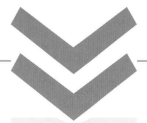

ASSISTED PULLUP

STRENGTHENS

LATS (BACK), BICEPS, SHOULDERS

STARTING POSITION

Grasp the assisted-pullup machine with a neutral grip (palms facing each other) and place your knees on the kneepad. Pull your shoulders back and down and lock in this position. Holding this position, simultaneously bring the other knee onto the pad as you lift up into the top starting position **(A)**.

MOVEMENT

Keeping your shoulders drawn inward, slowly lower your body until your arms are fully lengthened **(B)**. **EASY**

Immediately activate your back muscles and pull yourself upward to return to the starting position **(A)**. **HARD**

Pause at the top position before lowering.

Why It's Perfect for You

Traditional wide-grip pullups can be difficult to perform and they build wide backs.

The narrow neutral grip strengthens and tightens your back and core area from your underarm to your hip bone. It targets bra bulge under the arm and around the back, trouble zones for many women. Yay!

Alternative: Band-Assisted Pullup

If your gym doesn't have an assisted-pullup machine, you can get the same effect with a large circular workout rubber band and a pullup bar. Secure the band around the middle of the bar, allowing the other end to fall.

Grasp the bar with a neutral grip or palms-facing-you grip. Pull yourself up and slip your foot or knee onto the loop in the band. Keeping your shoulders drawn in, slowly lower yourself until your arms are straight. The band will stretch under your weight. The tension in the band will assist you as you do the pullup.

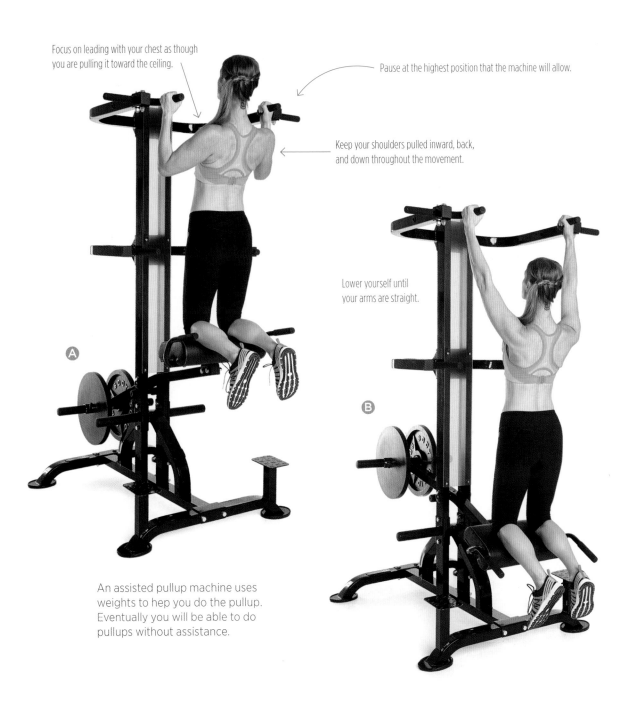

Focus on leading with your chest as though you are pulling it toward the ceiling.

Pause at the highest position that the machine will allow.

Keep your shoulders pulled inward, back, and down throughout the movement.

Lower yourself until your arms are straight.

A

B

An assisted pullup machine uses weights to hep you do the pullup. Eventually you will be able to do pullups without assistance.

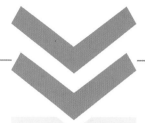

LYING DUMBBELL PULLOVER

STRENGTHENS

LATS (BACK), TRICEPS, CORE

STARTING POSITION

Lie on a flat bench with your feet up, holding one dumbbell with your arms extended. Keeping your abs contracted, allow a natural arch in your lower back. Push your shoulders down toward your hips (away from your ears) and against the bench **(A)**.

MOVEMENT

Keeping your shoulders locked in the starting position and your arms straight, slowly arc the dumbbell overhead, ending with your arms next to your ears **(B)**. **EASY**

Pause in this position.

Activate the muscles of your midback and triceps (back of your arms) to push the dumbbell back to the start **(A)**. **HARD**

Why It's Perfect for You

This move does triple duty. While it's primarily a back exercise, it also works your triceps and abs hard. It's amazing for tightening the backs of the arms and the flabby trouble zone around your bra strap.

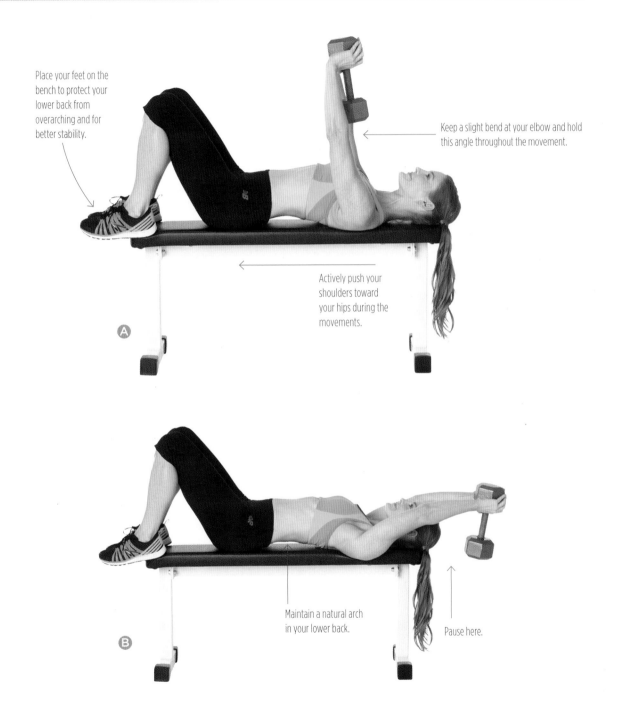

Place your feet on the bench to protect your lower back from overarching and for better stability.

Keep a slight bend at your elbow and hold this angle throughout the movement.

Actively push your shoulders toward your hips during the movements.

Ⓐ

Maintain a natural arch in your lower back.

Pause here.

Ⓑ

SEATED UPRIGHT CHEST FLY

STRENGTHENS

CHEST, ARMS, SHOULDERS

STARTING POSITION

Position the seat of the chest fly machine so that the handles are at the height of your chest. Grasp the handles and bring your hands together in front of your chest. Actively push your shoulders down toward your hips, away from your ears. Allow a natural arch in your lower back **(A)**.

MOVEMENT

Keeping your shoulders pressed down and your chest lifted, allow your arms to open outward. Keep a slight bend and constant angle at your elbow **(B)**. **EASY**

Pause in the open position with your hands in line with your chest at your sides (see inset).

Contract your chest muscles and bring your hands back together to the starting position **(A)**. **HARD**

Why It's Perfect for You

This movement strengthens your chest in a way that minimizes outward development and creates a very flattering décolleté, enhancing shape and cleavage in the chest. While this is primarily a chest exercise, it also makes women's biceps look great.

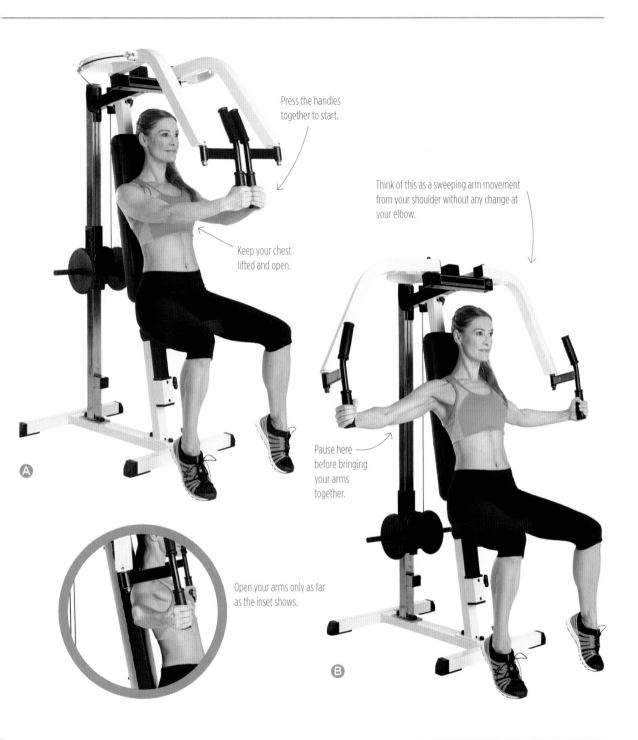

Press the handles together to start.

Think of this as a sweeping arm movement from your shoulder without any change at your elbow.

Keep your chest lifted and open.

Pause here before bringing your arms together.

Open your arms only as far as the inset shows.

Ⓐ

Ⓑ

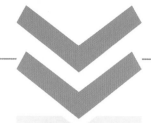

INCLINE DUMBBELL PRESS

STRENGTHENS

CHEST, SHOULDERS, TRICEPS

STARTING POSITION

Bring two dumbbells together over your chest while lying on a bench that is adjusted to a 45-degree incline. Extend your arms toward the ceiling, perpendicular to the floor, with your elbows unlocked. Allow a natural arch in your lower back **(A)**.

MOVEMENT

Pushing your shoulders down toward your hips (away from your ears) and against the bench, bend your elbows and open your arms outward **(B)**. **EASY**

Pause with the dumbbells over your elbows, near 90 degrees and directly out from your sides.

Contract your chest muscles and push the dumbbells back to the start **(A)**. **HARD**

Why It's Perfect for You

Women tend to be disproportionately weak in the chest. This movement strengthens the chest while also tightening up the triceps. It creates nice muscle definition in the front of the shoulders, making you look amazing in a strapless dress.

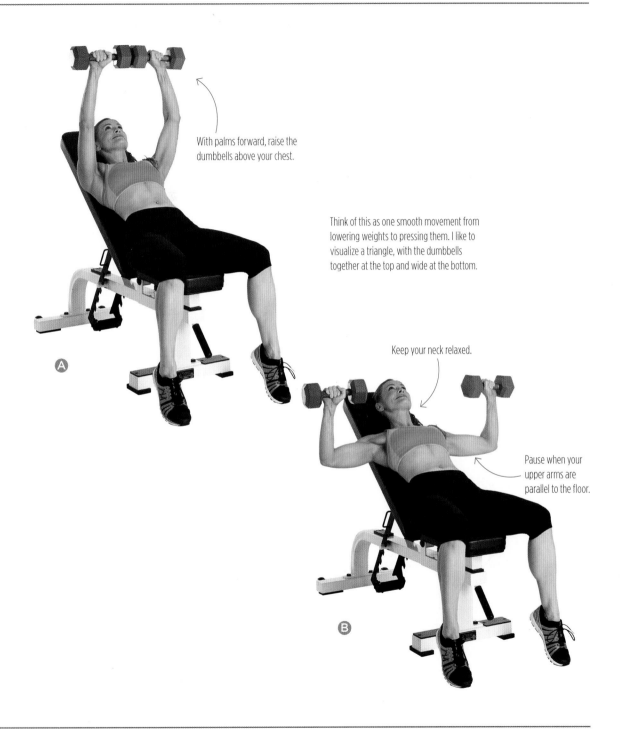

With palms forward, raise the dumbbells above your chest.

Think of this as one smooth movement from lowering weights to pressing them. I like to visualize a triangle, with the dumbbells together at the top and wide at the bottom.

Keep your neck relaxed.

Pause when your upper arms are parallel to the floor.

(A)

(B)

FLAT BENCH PRESS

Why It's Perfect for You

This might be the best overall chest strengthener of all. It is also a great foundation for many other movements and activities. This will improve your push-ups and chaturanga in yoga, while also targeting your triceps.

STRENGTHENS

CHEST, SHOULDERS, TRICEPS

STARTING POSITION

Using a full-length Olympic bar, lie on the bench with your feet up and your hands placed wider than your shoulders. Unrack the bar and bring it directly over your chest with your arms fully extended and unlocked at the elbow. Actively depress your shoulders down toward your hips **(A)**.

MOVEMENT

Bend your arms and allow the bar to slowly lower toward your chest. Aim for the middle of your chest directly over your nipple line **(B)**. **EASY**

Pause with the bar just above your chest.

Activate your chest muscles and press the bar straight back to the start **(A)**. **HARD**

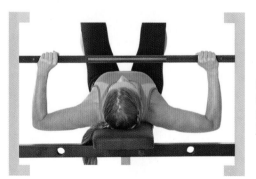

Look for the widest marks on the bar and place your hands so that your pinky finger is just inside this mark.

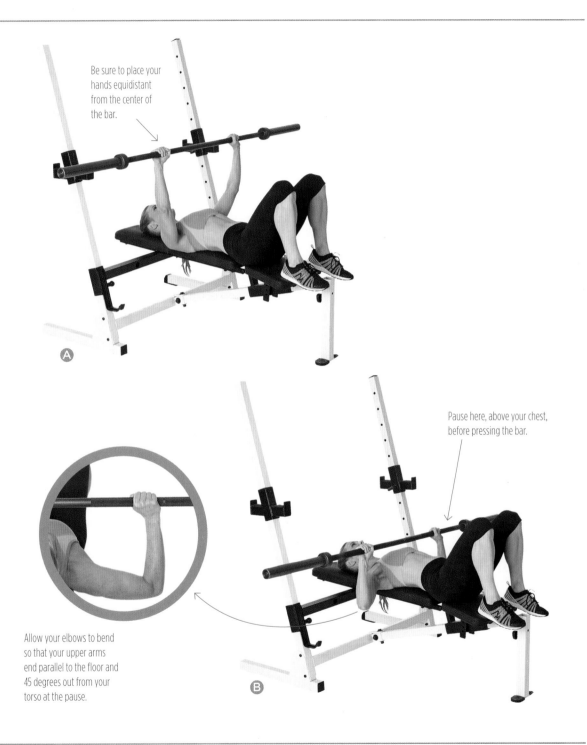

Be sure to place your hands equidistant from the center of the bar.

A

Pause here, above your chest, before pressing the bar.

B

Allow your elbows to bend so that your upper arms end parallel to the floor and 45 degrees out from your torso at the pause.

FLAT DUMBBELL FLY

Why It's Perfect for You

This move improves your chest strength without building muscle outward. It tones and tightens the area around your bra band as well as your arms. You'll create nice definition across your chest and eliminate any unwanted bulges around your bra straps.

STRENGTHENS

CHEST, SHOULDERS, ARMS

STARTING POSITION

Lie on a flat bench with your feet up and hold dumbbells together directly over your chest using a neutral grip (palms facing each other). Press your shoulders down toward your hips, and allow a natural arch in your lower back **(A)**.

MOVEMENT

Keeping a constant bend in your elbows, allow your arms to open outward in line with the middle of your chest **(B)**. **EASY**

Pause with your upper arms parallel to the floor and your hands in line with your chest.

Contract your chest muscles and arc the dumbbells back to the start with your palms facing each other **(A)**. **HARD**

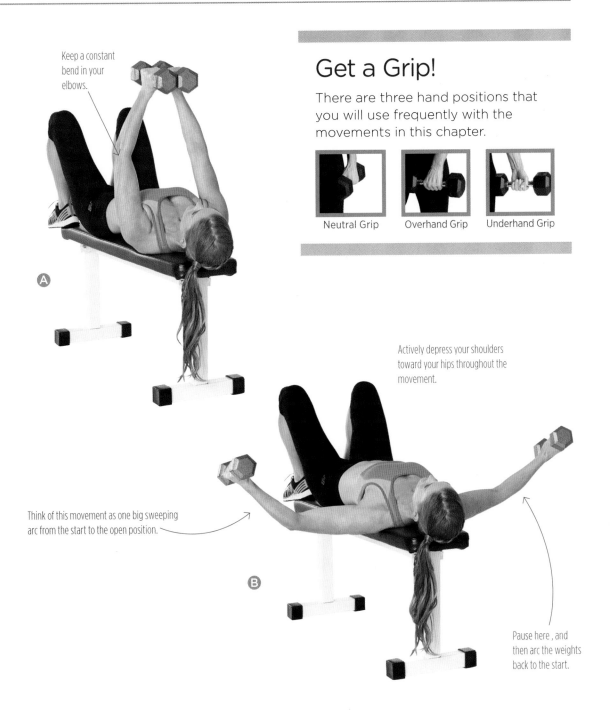

Keep a constant bend in your elbows.

A

Get a Grip!

There are three hand positions that you will use frequently with the movements in this chapter.

Neutral Grip Overhand Grip Underhand Grip

Actively depress your shoulders toward your hips throughout the movement.

Think of this movement as one big sweeping arc from the start to the open position.

B

Pause here , and then arc the weights back to the start.

BARBELL OVERHEAD PRESS

STRENGTHENS

SHOULDERS, TRICEPS

STARTING POSITION

Adjust the bench to a fully upright seated position. Grasp a shorter barbell with your hands slightly wider than your shoulders and press it into the overhead position. (You may need to ask spotters to hand the bar to you.) Release your shoulders down toward your hips while your arms are fully extended but not locked at the elbow. Maintain a slight arch in your lower back **(A)**.

MOVEMENT

Allow your arms to bend so that your elbows rotate forward and end directly below your hands with the bar in front of your collarbone **(B)**. **EASY**

Pause with the bar in this position.

Press the bar up, bypassing your face, and then arc backward to end directly over your head **(A)**. **HARD** See inset.

Why It's Perfect for You

Tank top alert! Nearly every client of mine wants definition in the front of the shoulders. This movement does it and makes your arms look amazing! The overhead pressing movement is really important for overall upper-body strength.

By supporting your body and back in a seated position, you are better able to focus your energy on the movement. Standing exercises disperse energy, making it harder to focus on the task at hand. Sitting also minimizes overusing your lower back during the Hard phase.

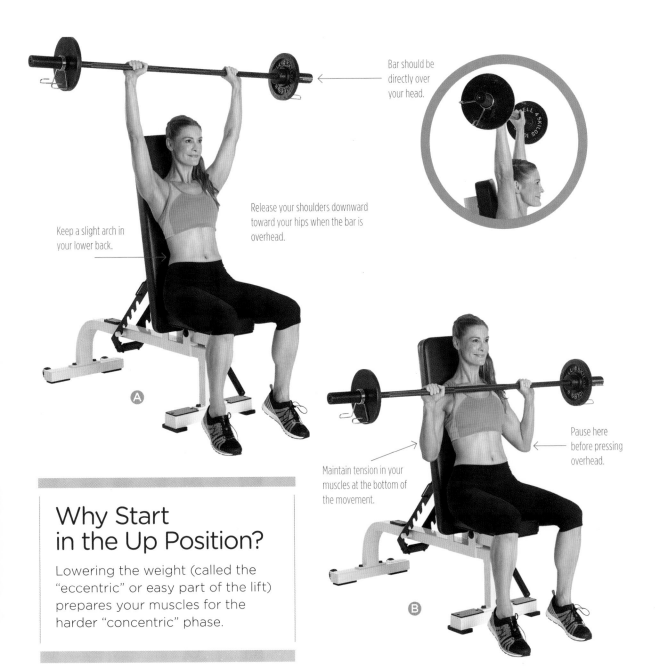

Bar should be directly over your head.

Keep a slight arch in your lower back.

Release your shoulders downward toward your hips when the bar is overhead.

A

Maintain tension in your muscles at the bottom of the movement.

Pause here before pressing overhead.

B

Why Start in the Up Position?

Lowering the weight (called the "eccentric" or easy part of the lift) prepares your muscles for the harder "concentric" phase.

DUMBBELL BENT ARM SIDE RAISE

STRENGTHENS

SHOULDERS (DELTOIDS), TRAPS

STARTING POSITION

Stand, holding dumbbells, with your feet together and your arms bent at your sides so that your elbows create a 90-degree angle. This means that the dumbbells are directly in front of your elbows **(A)**.

MOVEMENT

Keeping your shoulders pressed down toward your hips, maintain a constant angle at your elbows and raise your arms out to the sides and up **(B)**. **HARD**

Pause at the top with your arms parallel to the floor. Do this exercise in front of a mirror to make sure the dumbbells are positioned so that you cannot see your elbows.

Keeping your elbow angle the same, lower your arms back to the start **(A)**. **EASY**

Why It's Perfect for You

By performing this movement with your arms bent, you are better able to work against gravity to create roundness and definition in your shoulders.

Strength training is all about working against gravity. When your arms are in the straight position, they create a longer lever. This means that it is harder to get from point A to point B at any given weight. So a straight arm would require using lighter weights and therefore may not overload the deltoids sufficiently.

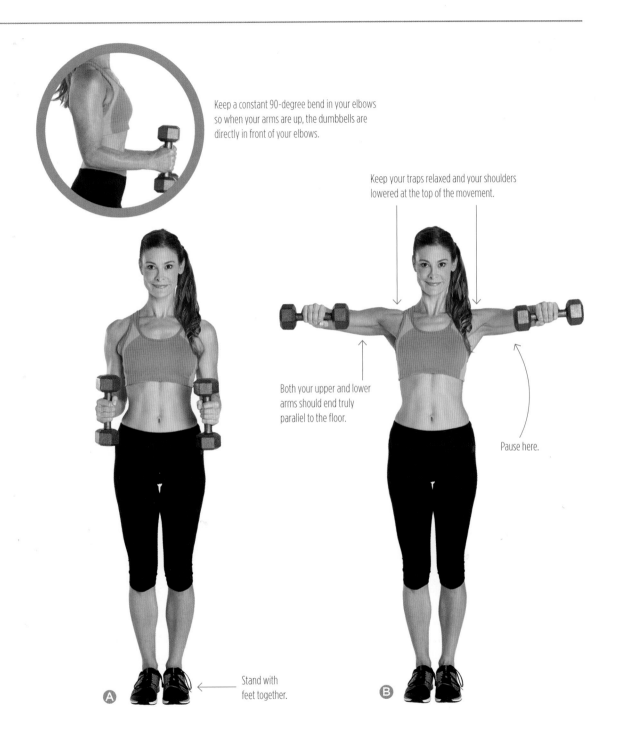

Keep a constant 90-degree bend in your elbows so when your arms are up, the dumbbells are directly in front of your elbows.

Keep your traps relaxed and your shoulders lowered at the top of the movement.

Both your upper and lower arms should end truly parallel to the floor.

Pause here.

Stand with feet together.

A

B

DUMBBELL UPRIGHT ROW

STRENGTHENS

SHOULDERS (DELTOIDS), TRAPS

STARTING POSITION

Stand with your feet separated by 2 to 4 inches, holding dumbbells in an overhand grip in front of your thighs. Keep your knees unlocked, and allow a natural arch in your lower back **(A)**.

MOVEMENT

Row the dumbbells in a direct upward line toward your shoulders, leading with your elbows. **HARD**

Pause very briefly at the top, ending with your elbows slightly higher than your shoulders and dumbbells directly in front of your shoulders. Allow the shoulders to elevate upward just a tiny bit **(B)**.

Slowly lower the weights to the start with dumbbells in front of your thighs **(A)**. **EASY**

Why It's Perfect for You

I like this dumbbell version of an upright row because it allows your arms and shoulders to move independently and more naturally compared to a barbell version. You can make small adjustments in your hand placement at the top to ensure sufficient pressure in your muscles. This movement creates an awesome fullness in your deltoid muscle, making your entire arm look more defined. While it's primarily a shoulder exercise, it also makes your biceps look great.

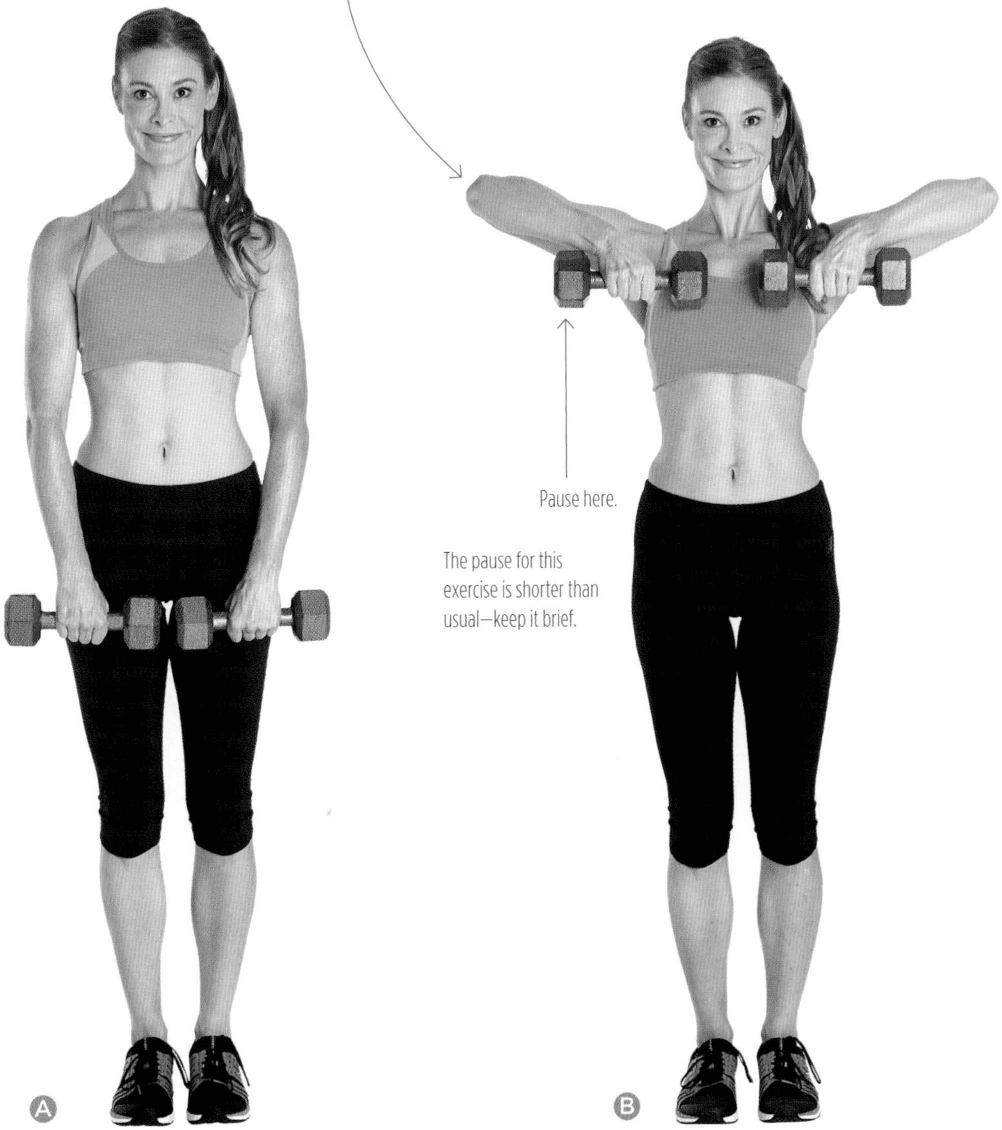

Think of this as an elbow-leading exercise rather than an arm movement. Use a mirror to ensure that your forearms end at an angle with your elbows higher than your shoulders.

Pause here.

The pause for this exercise is shorter than usual—keep it brief.

Use lightweight dumbbells for this exercise.

Ⓐ

Ⓑ

REVERSE DUMBBELL FLY

STRENGTHENS

SHOULDERS (POSTERIOR DELTOIDS), UPPER BACK

STARTING POSITION

Sit on a bench with your feet together at a 30-degree forward bend from your hips. Keep your arms extended with your elbows unlocked and your shoulders back and down toward your hips, allowing the dumbbells to hang down naturally below your shoulders **(A)**. Maintain a slight arch in your lower back throughout the movement.

MOVEMENT

With a natural upward movement from your torso, open your arms outward with very little change in your elbow angle **(B)**. **HARD**

Pause at the top with your shoulders contracted back and your arms at shoulder height.

Slowly lower your arms back to the start, returning to a 30-degree bend **(A)**. **EASY**

Why It's Perfect for You

This is an incredibly important exercise for optimal shoulder function and injury prevention. Beyond that, it makes the back of your shoulders look great and targets the trouble zone in the back of the arms by strengthening the upper region of your triceps. You'll also get rid of bra bulge under the arm and around the back.

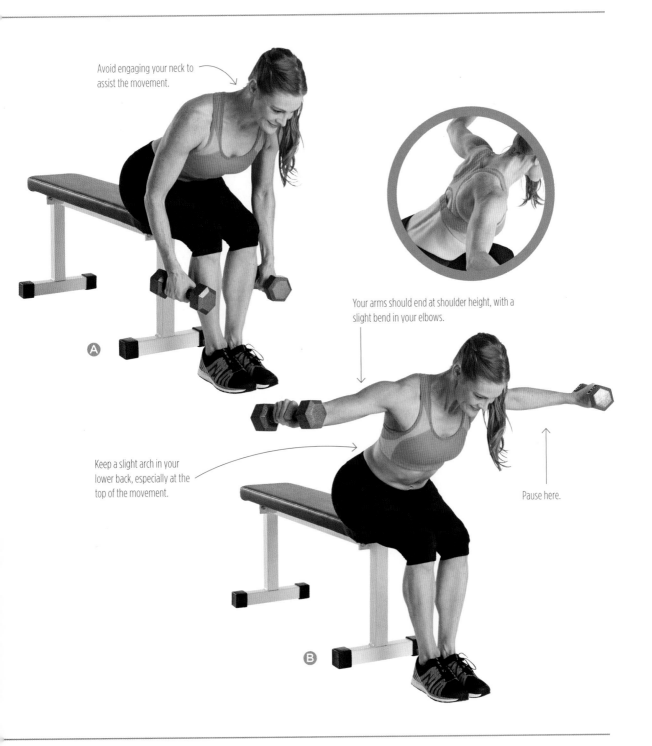

Avoid engaging your neck to assist the movement.

A

Keep a slight arch in your lower back, especially at the top of the movement.

Your arms should end at shoulder height, with a slight bend in your elbows.

Pause here.

B

STRAIGHT BAR CABLE PRESSDOWN

STRENGTHENS

TRICEPS

STARTING POSITION

Begin by facing the cable column with an overhand grip (palms facing down) on the short straight bar attachment. Stand with your feet together and your arms extended. Press the bar down so that your hands and the bar are touching your thighs. Draw your shoulders back and down, lift your chest, and maintain a slight arch in your lower back **(A)**.

MOVEMENT

Without moving your upper arms, bend your elbows until the bar ends in front of your chest **(B)**. **EASY**

Pause in this position without releasing your shoulders.

Contract the back of your arms to press the bar back to the start, ending with your elbows nearly locked and the bar touching your thighs **(A)**. **HARD**

Why It's Perfect for You

I love the way the straight bar targets the back of your arms. This is by far my favorite triceps exercise because it's so effective. It emphasizes the upper region of your triceps, which tend to be weak and underworked.

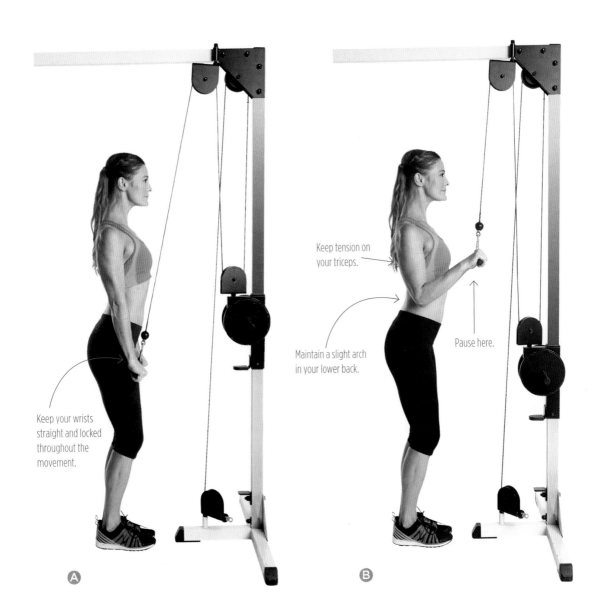

Keep tension on
your triceps.

Maintain a slight arch
in your lower back.

Pause here.

Keep your wrists
straight and locked
throughout the
movement.

Ⓐ

Ⓑ

DUMBBELL FRENCH PRESS

STRENGTHENS

TRICEPS

STARTING POSITION

Lie on a flat bench with your feet up and dumbbells extended together directly over your chest in a neutral grip (palms facing each other). Allow a natural arch in your lower back, and actively press your shoulders down toward your hips **(A)**.

MOVEMENT

Without changing the position of your hands, bend your elbows and slowly lower the dumbbells next to your ears **(B)**. **EASY**

Pause with the dumbbells next to your ears.

Activate your triceps to push the dumbbells back to the start, ending with nearly locked elbows **(A)**. **HARD**

Why It's Perfect for You

This is the perfect complement to the last exercise, the Straight Bar Cable Pressdown, because of the hand position. This movement targets the triceps and creates definition in the middle of your upper arm. By anchoring your shoulders down toward your hips, you also improve shoulder stability.

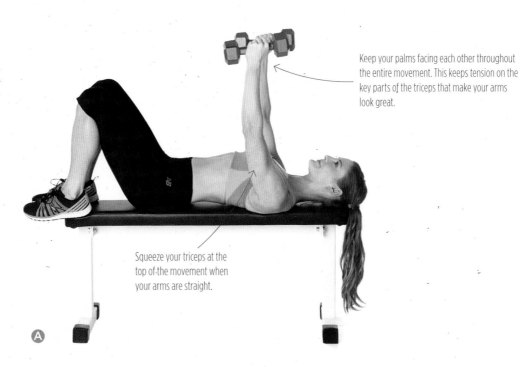

Keep your palms facing each other throughout the entire movement. This keeps tension on the key parts of the triceps that make your arms look great.

Squeeze your triceps at the top of the movement when your arms are straight.

A

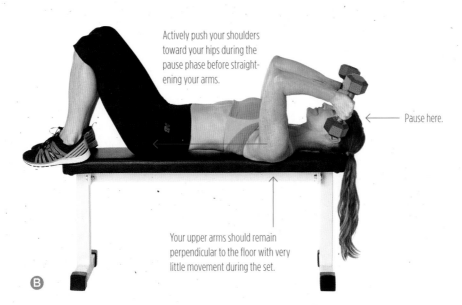

Actively push your shoulders toward your hips during the pause phase before straightening your arms.

Pause here.

Your upper arms should remain perpendicular to the floor with very little movement during the set.

B

OVERHEAD ROPE EXTENSION

STRENGTHENS

TRICEPS, SHOULDER STABILIZERS

STARTING POSITION

Using the double-rope attachment, face away from the cable column in a staggered foot stance. Extend your arms outward until they are straight with nearly locked elbows. Anchor your shoulders down toward your hips and maintain this position **(A)**.

MOVEMENT

Without changing the angle of your upper arm, allow your elbows to bend so that your hands move over your head toward the cable column **(B)**. **EASY**

Pause with your elbows bent around 90 degrees.

Activate your triceps to drive your arms back to the starting position with elbows nearly locked **(A)**. **HARD**

Why It's Perfect for You

I love how this movement keeps tension on the triceps, allowing for more time to build strong arms. It also helps to improve shoulder stability and to eliminate bra bulge under the arm and around the back, trouble zones for many women.

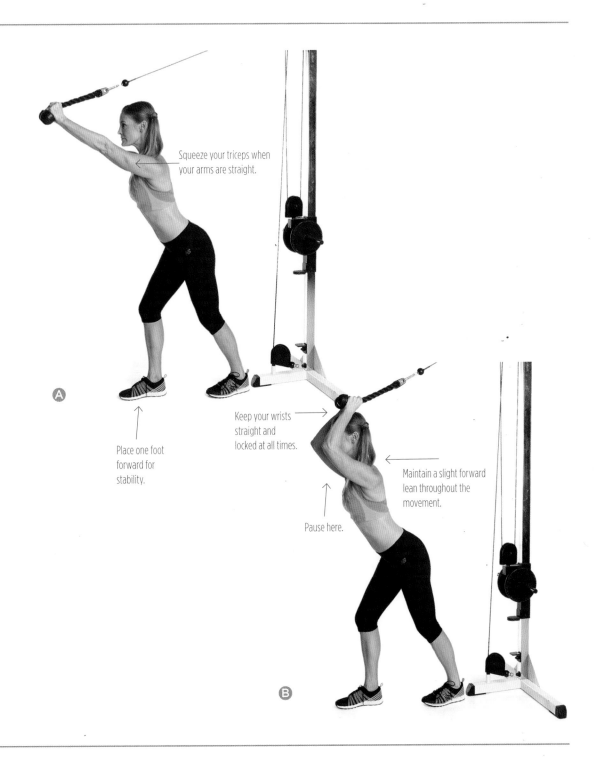

Squeeze your triceps when your arms are straight.

A

Place one foot forward for stability.

Keep your wrists straight and locked at all times.

Maintain a slight forward lean throughout the movement.

Pause here.

B

● TRICEPS

ALTERNATIVE: ROPE PRESSDOWN

STRENGTHENS

TRICEPS

STARTING POSITION

Using the double-rope attachment, face the cable column with your feet together, knees slightly bent, a natural arch in your lower back, and your shoulders back and down. Press the rope down so that your arms begin straight with your hands separated as much as possible. Allow a slight bend in your wrists in this position **(A)**.

MOVEMENT

Keeping your shoulders anchored down, slowly bend your elbows, keeping your upper arms perpendicular to the floor **(B)**. **EASY**

Pause with your elbows bent and forearms just above parallel to the floor.

Activate your triceps to press the rope down to the starting position with your hands separated **(A)**. **HARD**

Why It's Perfect for You

This is a great alternative to the previous movement, the Overhead Rope Extension. This movement has less time under tension but allows for greater attention on the upper region of your triceps. This option is great if you don't love the staggered stance or overhead position of the Overhead Rope Extension or if you have any shoulder issues.

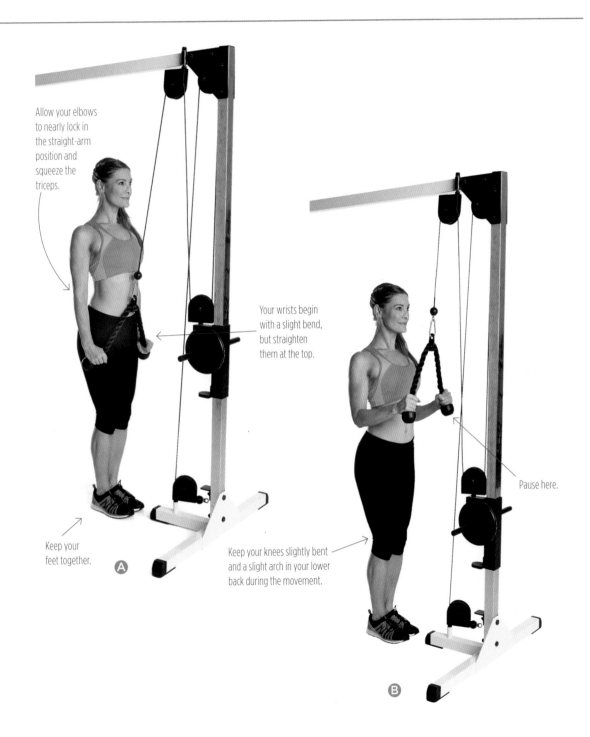

Allow your elbows to nearly lock in the straight-arm position and squeeze the triceps.

Your wrists begin with a slight bend, but straighten them at the top.

Keep your feet together.

Ⓐ

Pause here.

Keep your knees slightly bent and a slight arch in your lower back during the movement.

Ⓑ

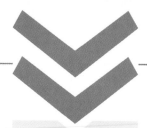

DUMBBELL HAMMER CURL

STRENGTHENS

BICEPS, SHOULDERS (ANTERIOR DELTOIDS)

STARTING POSITION

Begin in a seated position with dumbbells hanging at your sides in a neutral grip (palms facing each other). Sit tall with your chest forward and your shoulders back and down **(A)**.

MOVEMENT

Without changing your hand position, contract your biceps and pull the dumbbells up until the ends nearly touch the front of your shoulders **(B)**. **HARD**

Pause in this position and squeeze your biceps.

Keeping your shoulders anchored down and back, slowly lower the dumbbells back to the start **(A)**. **EASY**

Why It's Perfect for You

This particular hand position makes for amazing definition and roundedness in the front of the upper arm. The seated position lets you focus all energy on the movement.

Maintaining a neutral grip allows your muscle to develop in a narrow and rounded way, rather than creating thickness. Men like thick, full biceps and women tend to prefer rounded, thin biceps.

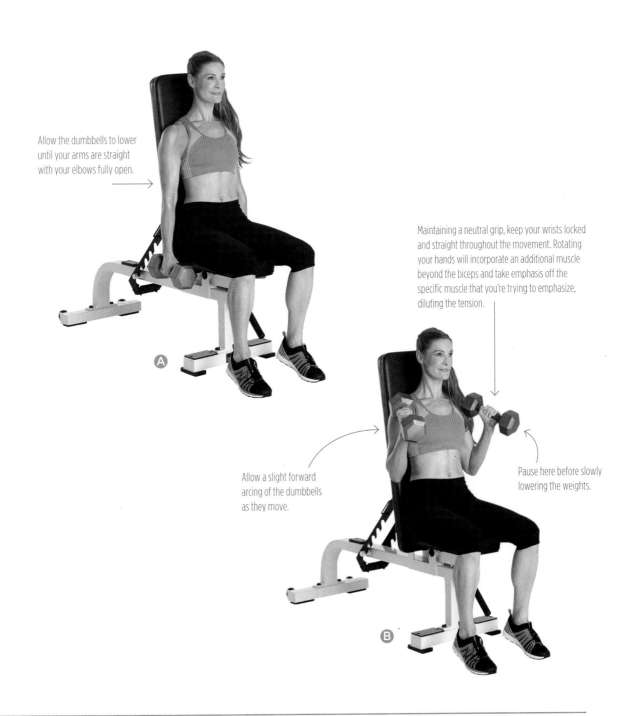

Allow the dumbbells to lower until your arms are straight with your elbows fully open.

Maintaining a neutral grip, keep your wrists locked and straight throughout the movement. Rotating your hands will incorporate an additional muscle beyond the biceps and take emphasis off the specific muscle that you're trying to emphasize, diluting the tension.

Allow a slight forward arcing of the dumbbells as they move.

Pause here before slowly lowering the weights.

A

B

STRAIGHT BAR CABLE CURL

STRENGTHENS

BICEPS

STARTING POSITION

Begin by facing the cable column with a supinated grip (palms facing out) on the short straight bar attachment. Keep your arms extended, your hands at shoulder-width distance, and your feet together. Stand tall with a natural arch in your lower back, your shoulders pulled back and down, and your chest forward **(A)**.

MOVEMENT

Bend at the elbows without moving your upper arms. Contracting your biceps, pull the bar up to your collarbone **(B)**. **HARD**

Pause in the top position, keeping tension on your biceps.

Keeping your upper arms perpendicular to the floor and your shoulders locked, slowly lower the bar back to the start **(A)**. **EASY**

Why It's Perfect for You

The *bi* in *biceps* indicates there are two "heads" to your upper arm muscles. This movement complements the previous exercise, the Dumbbell Hammer Curl, because each exercise addresses one head of the biceps. This movement makes the arm stronger, while the previous one creates shape and definition.

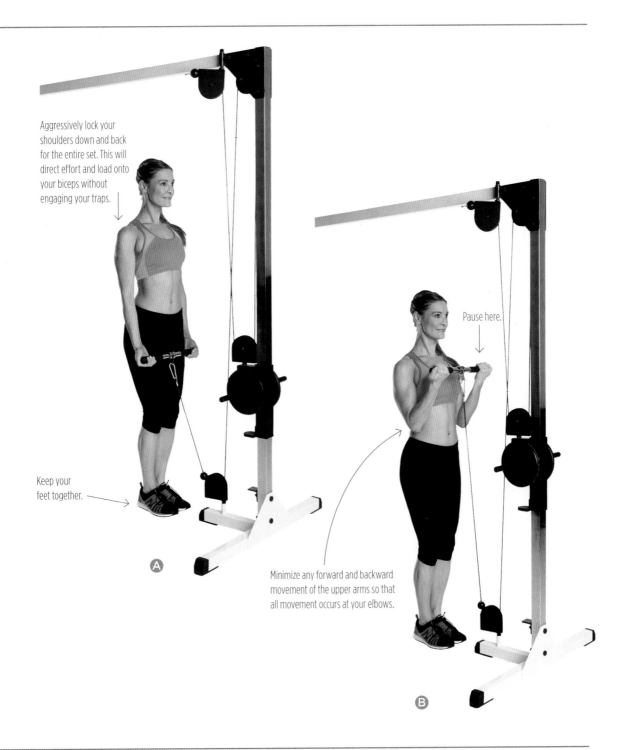

Aggressively lock your shoulders down and back for the entire set. This will direct effort and load onto your biceps without engaging your traps.

Pause here.

Keep your feet together.

Minimize any forward and backward movement of the upper arms so that all movement occurs at your elbows.

A

B

ALTERNATING DUMBBELL SUPINATED CURL

STRENGTHENS

BICEPS, SHOULDERS (ANTERIOR DELTOIDS)

STARTING POSITION

Stand with your feet together and dumbbells at your sides, touching your thighs, with your palms facing out (a supinated grip). Keep your knees unlocked and your shoulders pulled back and down **(A)**.

MOVEMENT

Without changing your hand position, pull the right dumbbell up to the front of your shoulder **(B)**. **HARD**

Pause here and squeeze the biceps muscles.

Maintaining your hand position, lower the dumbbell back to the start **EASY** while simultaneously pulling the left dumbbell up to the front of your shoulder **(C)**. **HARD**

Continue simultaneous alternating for the full set. One arm will be in the **HARD** phase, while the other will be in the **EASY** phase.

Why It's Perfect for You

Because you are simultaneously alternating, you will increase the pressure and intensity in your muscles by limiting rest time in between reps. This improves the time under tension and creates change. You'll feel an awesome "pump" after this exercise!

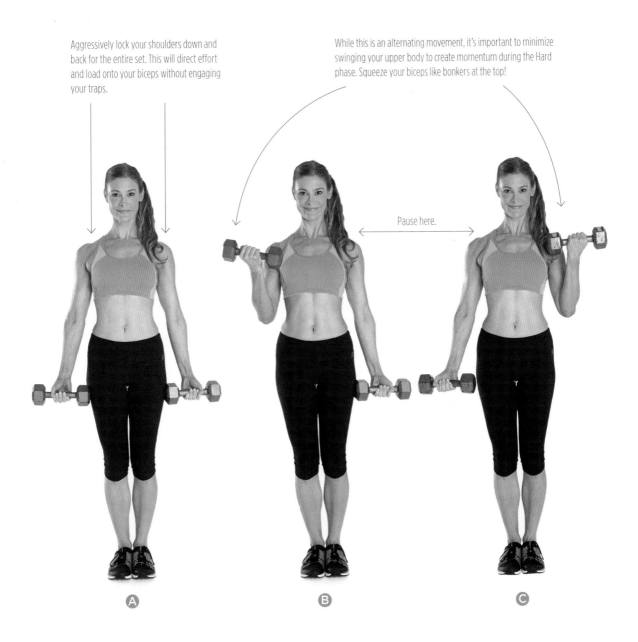

Aggressively lock your shoulders down and back for the entire set. This will direct effort and load onto your biceps without engaging your traps.

While this is an alternating movement, it's important to minimize swinging your upper body to create momentum during the Hard phase. Squeeze your biceps like bonkers at the top!

Pause here.

Ⓐ

Ⓑ

Ⓒ

ALL FOURS CRUNCH

STRENGTHENS

ABS (RECTUS ABDOMINIS, TRANSVERSUS ABDOMINIS)

STARTING POSITION

Lie on your back with your knees bent, feet flat, and hands resting behind your ears. Draw inward with your abs **(A)**.

MOVEMENT

Initiate action from your core and simultaneously bring your elbows and knees together, attempting to touch them above your navel **(B)**. **HARD**

Pause at the highest point and contract your abs deeply.

Slowly release, lowering your upper and lower body simultaneously, allowing your arms to return to the starting position in contact with the floor **(A)**. **EASY**

Why It's Perfect for You

This is a great basic movement that strengthens torso flexion. Crunch-type movements are valuable for both core contractibility and appearance as long as other core movements complement them. This is the only traditional crunch of the five core movements in this section.

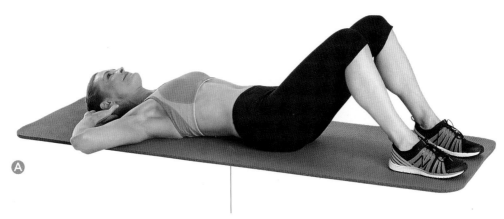

A

Do not flatten your lower back onto the floor. Think instead of drawing your abs inward. If you are unable to bring your elbows and knees to touch at the top, find an appropriate point to pause where you can get an effective "squeeze" without straining.

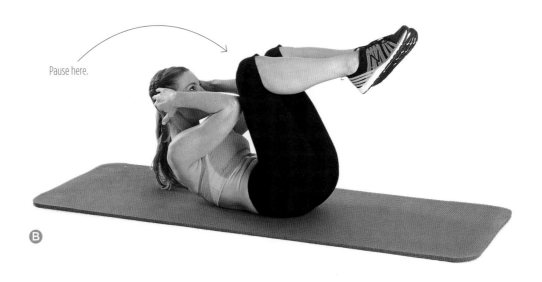

Pause here.

B

BICYCLE

STRENGTHENS

ALL FOUR AB MUSCLES THAT COLLECTIVELY FORM YOUR CORE

STARTING POSITION

Lie on the floor, contract your abs, and bring your elbows and knees together over your torso **(A)**.

MOVEMENT

Extend your left leg outward to a 45-degree angle from the floor, and bring your right knee in toward you. Simultaneously twist and bring your left elbow to your right knee **(B)**. **HARD**

Pause with your left elbow and right knee touching or as close as possible.

Keeping a contracted position with your shoulders off the floor, immediately switch your elbows and knees so that your right leg extends out and your left knee bends inward. Simultaneously cross your right elbow over to your left knee to complete the movement on the opposite side **(C)**. **HARD**

Continue alternating your elbows and knees for the entire set. This means that your torso stays in a contracted position with your shoulders off the floor for the whole set.

Why It's Perfect for You

This is the mack daddy of core movements because it incorporates all the major muscles of your torso. This move creates tightness with some definition, not rigid, sculpted, bodybuilder-style ab muscles. It also serves a very important functional purpose by strengthening the transversus abdominis muscle that supports your spine.

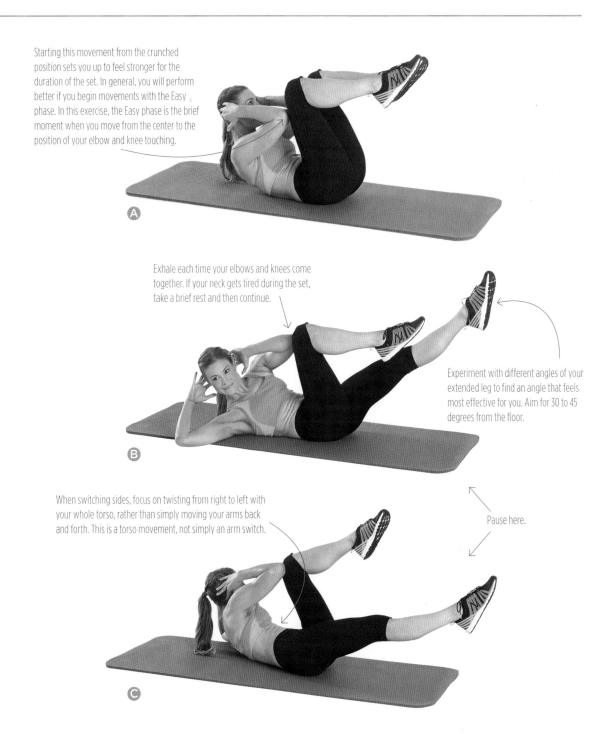

Starting this movement from the crunched position sets you up to feel stronger for the duration of the set. In general, you will perform better if you begin movements with the Easy phase. In this exercise, the Easy phase is the brief moment when you move from the center to the position of your elbow and knee touching.

A

Exhale each time your elbows and knees come together. If your neck gets tired during the set, take a brief rest and then continue.

Experiment with different angles of your extended leg to find an angle that feels most effective for you. Aim for 30 to 45 degrees from the floor.

B

When switching sides, focus on twisting from right to left with your whole torso, rather than simply moving your arms back and forth. This is a torso movement, not simply an arm switch.

Pause here.

C

WEIGHTED BALL FLEXION

STRENGTHENS

ABS (RECTUS ABDOMINIS, TRANSVERSUS ABDOMINIS)

STARTING POSITION

Using a 55- or 65-centimeter physioball, sit on the front quadrant, holding a weight plate across your chest **(A)**. See the inset for how to hold the plate.

MOVEMENT

From the upright seated position, engage your abs and slowly rotate backward as you allow the ball to counterrotate under you just a little bit **(B)**. **EASY**

Pause on the back end at the point where you feel solid pressure in your core, where you are balanced but not straining.

Squeeze your abs to pull yourself back up to the starting position **(A)**, allowing the ball to counterrotate back to the start. **HARD**

Why It's Perfect for You

This is one of the only weighted core exercises I like for most women. It's a great way to truly strengthen your core in a functional and aesthetic manner. It will make you stronger by forcing you to balance while you flex up and back.

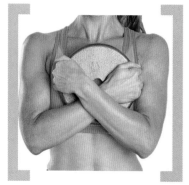

Hold the plate, 5 to 10 pounds, high on your chest.

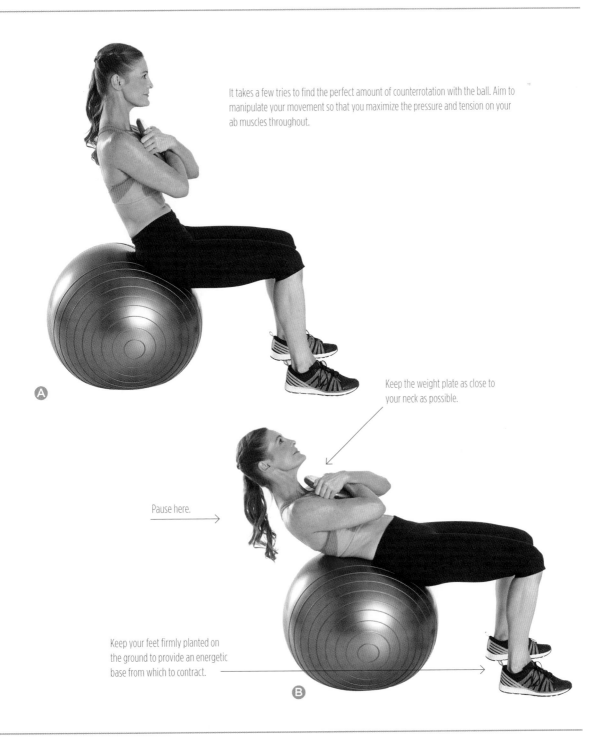

It takes a few tries to find the perfect amount of counterrotation with the ball. Aim to manipulate your movement so that you maximize the pressure and tension on your ab muscles throughout.

Keep the weight plate as close to your neck as possible.

Pause here.

Keep your feet firmly planted on the ground to provide an energetic base from which to contract.

PLANK ON BALL

STRENGTHENS

ABS (RECTUS ABDOMINIS, TRANSVERSUS ABDOMINIS)

STARTING POSITION

Using a 55- or 65-centimeter physioball, from your knees, place your elbows directly under your shoulders and clasp your hands. This is your foundation, so take your time to set this up strongly. Step back into a plank position with your feet 2 to 4 inches apart. Draw inward with your abs, but keep a natural curve in your lower back and avoid flattening it.

MOVEMENT

Hold this position for the time noted in your 90-day training program. You can either use a stopwatch or try your best to count it out in your head.

Why It's Perfect for You

This is the ultimate functional exercise for core stability and spine support. Its origin is from the world of physical therapy, and it is very important for alignment.

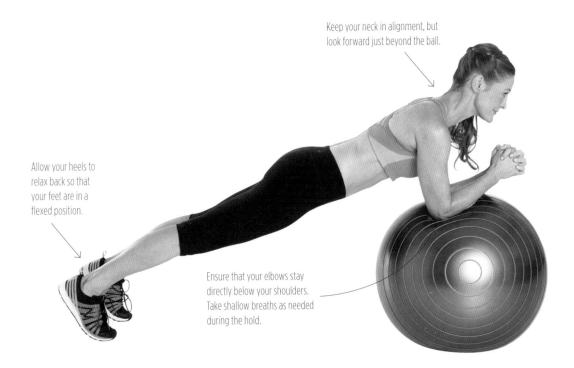

Keep your neck in alignment, but look forward just beyond the ball.

Allow your heels to relax back so that your feet are in a flexed position.

Ensure that your elbows stay directly below your shoulders. Take shallow breaths as needed during the hold.

HANGING KNEE-UP

STRENGTHENS

ABS AND CORE, SHOULDER GIRDLE

STARTING POSITION

Using the captain's chair, prop yourself high with your elbows under your shoulders. Aggressively reach your head up toward the ceiling to maintain an energetic lift **(A)**. This creates the ideal foundation from your shoulder girdle.

MOVEMENT

Bring your knees forward and upward by contracting your abs and without using momentum **(B)**. **HARD**

Pause with your knees at chest height. Your pelvis should tuck under and pull away from the pad just a tiny bit.

Slowly lower your legs back to a straightened, hanging position **(A)**. **EASY**

Why It's Perfect for You

This. Will. Make. You. STRONG.

While this exercise is for your abs and core, there is a secondary benefit that comes from propping yourself up in the chair. By aggressively extending upward, you will be pushing with the muscles at the base of your shoulder blades. This improves shoulder-girdle stability. Also, the action of extending toward the ceiling strengthens the area under the arm and around the back that causes bra bulge.

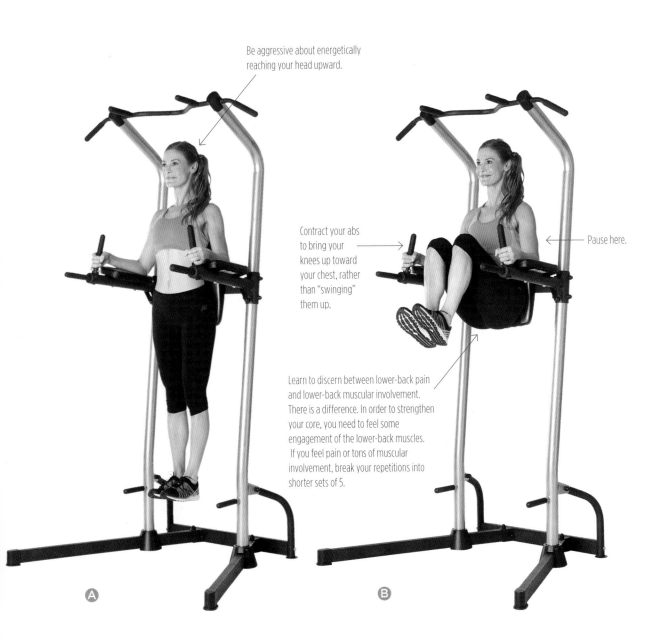

Be aggressive about energetically reaching your head upward.

Contract your abs to bring your knees up toward your chest, rather than "swinging" them up.

Pause here.

Learn to discern between lower-back pain and lower-back muscular involvement. There is a difference. In order to strengthen your core, you need to feel some engagement of the lower-back muscles. If you feel pain or tons of muscular involvement, break your repetitions into shorter sets of 5.

A

B

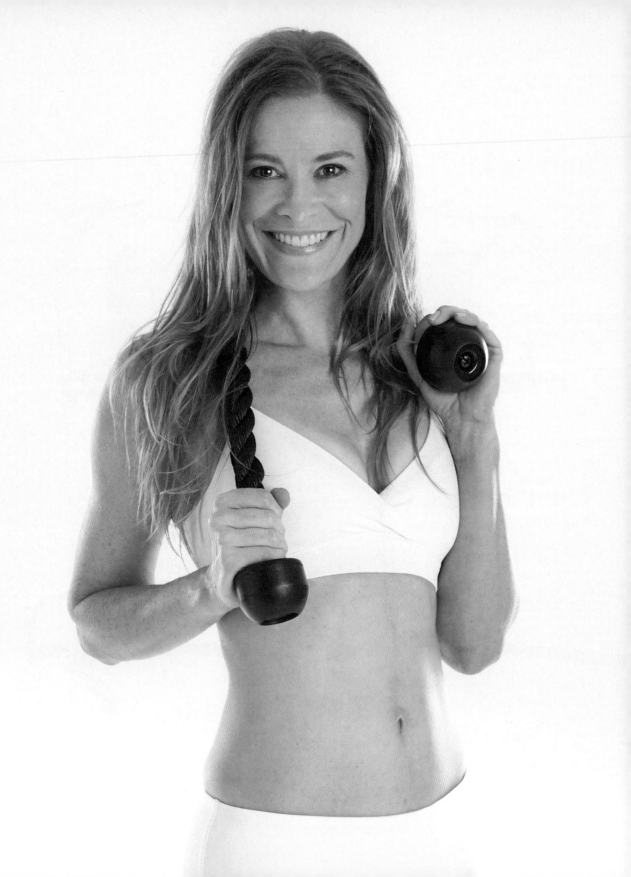

Part III
Your 90-Day Training Programs

Lift
to Get
Lean

Chapter 8
How to Pick Your Ideal 90-Day Training Program

The four training programs in this book are all 90 days. If 90 days seems daunting to you, think of it as 12 weeks, or 3 months. It's a silly game I play with myself all the time. Three months just sounds easier, right?

Let's stop for a moment and do one of my favorite visualization exercises. I want you to visualize your body in the form that you deeply desire. If I could swoop in and wave my magic Holly wand and turn you into the fitness queen you've always wanted to be, what would you look like? Visualize it in your mind, imagining that you are looking into a mirror at yourself. When you see the reflection of you in peak shape, what do you see? Do you see full, rounded shoulders? Do you see sculpted, defined arms and a solid and strong midsection? Do you see a happier, more energized version of yourself?

In addition, I want you to experience how you'd feel if you achieved this body that you are visualizing. How would you feel—physically, emotionally,

You Cannot Fail If You Do This One Thing

The one fail-proof strategy? Be consistent. If you eat fast food 6 days a week and then binge on kale, salmon, and berries for 1 day, you'll never see the benefits of that 1-day splurge on healthy foods. But flip that around—eat healthy for 6 days a week and then splurge on pizza or hamburgers for 1 day—and you probably will. Same goes for strength training. Your body is designed to survive and maintain its homeostasis, its physiological comfort zone. Therefore, your body will only change when you expose it to something new consistently. This is particularly true when it comes to changing the female body. Because building muscle is inherently against our genetics, it takes some time to create real and lasting change. It also takes some time for your body to make the necessary adaptations that cause an increase in lean muscle mass and a decrease in body fat. If you feel your motivation waning after a few weeks, make yourself stick with it. Radical change takes time—but the results are worth it. The only way you'll fail is if you give up. Don't!

spiritually? What exactly does it feel like to be leaner and tighter than you have ever been? Sometimes during exercises like this there's a part of your brain that chimes in whispering words of judgment. For this exercise, make a conscious effort to dismiss any critical language or negative thinking that might come up. For today, just focus on all of the wonderful things you see and feel when you look in the mirror at "You 2.0."

So go ahead and have fun with this visualization exercise. Take 1 or 2 minutes right now and deeply connect to this image of yourself in the mirror. Close your eyes and breathe. I'll still be here when you come back. Go.

Awesome, right? Were you able to dismiss those evil negative voices? Were you able to see the newly cultivated strength and vitality in your body? What emotions did you feel? Pride? Accomplishment? Empowerment? Did you feel like you wanted to holler "Yay me!"?

Now ask yourself again if you really believe that 3 months is a "long time" to finally realize this full potential. It's not. Ninety days is all it takes to make radical, life-altering changes in your body. You can do this. And you're worth it.

Pick Your Plan

Nearly all women fall into one of four broad fitness categories. These categories take into consideration things like how you produce energy, how your muscles respond to strength training, and how your hormonal profile influences your body composition.

Most fitness books offer only one general program. This is inherently flawed. Because our bodies, experience levels, and preferences are all very different, you need a program that's right for you. After all, how many times has a one-size-fits-all T-shirt actually fit you?

The 90-day training programs in this book address the needs of each fitness category with different workouts and strategies. But each program is designed to create the same ideal outcome: your body in a stronger, leaner, more powerful form.

The four programs are:

1. Newbie
2. Easy Gainer
3. Hard Gainer
4. Radical Transformation

Each of the four programs targets every major muscle group in your body. Every plan will also:

> Improve your overall strength
> Increase your lean muscle mass
> Improve the balance and symmetry between your muscle groups
> Supercharge your metabolism
> Naturally decrease your body fat
> Create a visually stunning feminine physique
> Create a strong sense of inner strength and resilience

The key to finding the right program is to choose the one that best reflects your current situation. Take a moment and ask yourself the following questions.

Do you have at least 6 months of consistent experience strength training?

Answer, then consider . . .

YES	**NO**
Easy Gainer, Hard Gainer, or Radical Transformation	Newbie or Easy Gainer

Are you time-crunched? Do you need to limit your number of workouts per week?

Answer, then consider . . .

YES	**NO**
Newbie or Easy Gainer	Newbie, Easy Gainer, Hard Gainer, or Radical Transformation

From experience, do you know for certain that you tend to build muscle easily?

Answer, then consider . . .

YES	**NO**
Easy Gainer	Easy Gainer, Newbie, Hard Gainer, or Radical Transformation

Have you been unsuccessful at getting lean despite regular strength workouts?

Answer, then consider . . .

YES	**NO**
Hard Gainer or Radical Transformation	Easy Gainer or Radical Transformation

Are you lifting weights regularly but still a bit confused?

Answer, then consider . . .

YES	**NO**
Newbie or Hard Gainer	Hard Gainer or Radical Transformation

Are you an established fitness enthusiast interested in radically changing your body and fitness level?

Answer, then consider . . .

YES	**NO**
Radical Transformation	Newbie, Easy Gainer, or Hard Gainer

If there's one program that already stands out to you, trust your gut—that's probably the right plan for you. If you're undecided, browse through the next few chapters for more details about each program.

Are You a Little Nervous Right Now?

So, are you a little scared about stepping into the weights section of your gym and taking your program for a spin? If you're anything like me, you get apprehensive about new activities. It took me a long time to figure out that source of the butterflies is the unknown.

Whenever I am faced with doing something new, I think of this quote: "Fear is excitement with the brakes on." And it's a very human feeling.

It's time for you to ease up on the brakes and embrace the fun. You've got something to be excited about. Stepping out of your comfort zone and into the gym is going to make you grow in ways that are hard to explain until you've experienced them. Take a deep breath and remember: It might be unfamiliar and unknown, but you can't make a mistake. This journey into strength training is going to be so rewarding and is worth drumming up some courage for.

Chapter 9
Newbie

This is a simplified and time-efficient program that is thorough and effective in just two workouts per week. I call this plan "Newbie," but it's not only for beginners. Whether you're a true weight-lifting novice or you're coming off of an extended break, this program will give you a solid strength-training foundation.

If you're new to lifting weights, it provides just the right amount of stimulus to create a lean body, but it isn't too much for your untrained system. If you are just beginning your strength-training journey, it's important to begin somewhat slowly and not overtax your muscles to avoid soreness. The human body does better with slow and gradual increases in fitness demands.

Newbie is also great if you are experienced in the gym but need a reboot of sorts. If you are returning to the gym after a hiatus, or want to relearn the basics, Newbie is perfect for you. (Don't be put off by the name. Even experienced athletes go back to the basics to build foundational strength every now and then.)

This plan uses the fewest exercises, which is intentional. I remember feeling overwhelmed when I started to explore strength-based workouts many years ago. Even though I had an advanced education in fitness, I still got very intimidated when I would enter the weights section of my gym. There were so many different machines, with knobs and buttons and pulleys and all sorts of whatnot. Eventually I decided that I would make better progress if I started with just one or two machines and focused on those until I mastered them. This is a philosophy that still holds true for me to this day. I'm a big believer in taking baby steps, because *anything* is better than nothing. If something overwhelms me, I tend to back off rather than dive in—and so do many people (even smart, accomplished ones). This program teaches foundation movements that should be mastered before moving on to more complex exercises.

Newbie is right for you if you are:

> Just beginning your strength-training journey
> Returning to exercise after a prolonged hiatus
> Ready to begin the rehab process after an injury
> Limited on time and desire a "bare minimum" workout for strength
> Trying to master basic movement patterns to build a foundation for more advanced training

You should begin with Newbie if it reflects your *current* situation. You will see better results faster if you work with your body's current abilities. Your body will respond best if you challenge it only 20 percent beyond its current ability. If you attempt too much too soon, your body will find sneaky ways to sabotage your fitness efforts.

If one of the five bullets above applies to you, start with this program. Once your body has sufficiently adapted to the exercises, you can revisit this book and follow the Radical Transformation program.

How the Plan Works

Newbie is a full-body program divided up into two workouts per week. Each workout will take you approximately 25 to 35 minutes to complete and targets four major muscle groups. Workout A targets your legs, back, biceps, and abs. Workout B targets your legs, chest, triceps, and shoulders.

Newbie Quick Look

Right for you if:
You are brand new
to strength training
or need a time-
efficient, bare-
minimum program.

**Workouts per
week:** 2
Full body: Yes!
Skill level:
Beginner to
Advanced
**Number of
exercises:** 16
Time per workout:
25–35 minutes

Your week at a glance: The ideal way to split up your weekly workouts for this program is to allow 2 days of rest in between Workout A and Workout B. This may seem like you're not working out that much, but it's important to allow sufficient time for recovery before stressing your muscles again.

Here's one way to schedule.

Monday: Workout A
Thursday: Workout B

Or if you prefer to exercise on a weekend, here's another option.

Wednesday: Workout A
Saturday: Workout B

The month-by-month progression: Because the legs represent over half of the body in general, it's important to strengthen them twice each week at a bare minimum. All other major muscle groups will get targeted once per week.

Month 1: You will complete two sets of each exercise with short rest periods and a moderate number of reps. This will allow your body to lay the foundation so that you can gradually ramp up the intensity a bit in the 2nd and 3rd months.

Month 2: You will see an increase in the number of sets or reps and get a slightly longer rest phase to help you recover from this extra work. This allows you to enter your next set strongly. The increase in sets and reps here is the progressive resistance (increased intensity over time) necessary to inspire progress.

Month 3: By now, you'll be feeling solid improvements in your strength and fitness level. So this is the month to really dig in and challenge your muscles to create more lean muscle mass that will supercharge your metabolism and burn off excess body fat. To do this, you'll be doing fewer reps but more sets overall compared to last month. Fewer reps means you'll be using heavier weights, so

How and When to Increase the Weight Load

The beauty of my Three-Step System to Strength is that it guides you through questions like this. If you are observing all three steps, you'll know when to increase your weight loads by the quality of the last 2 reps. If the last 2 reps of any set demonstrate perfect technique, you should increase your weight load for the next set. If the last 2 reps are less than perfect, you can feel confident in your weight load for each exercise.

In the program that follows, I've also specified very specific rest phases for each month. Because I give you longer rest phases each month, you'll be able to perform your exercises with heavier weight loads. This is one way that my programming helps to ensure your goals.

In general, the name of the game is to always be striving to perform every exercise at higher weight loads. Stay committed to the Last 2 Reps Rule and you'll always know when it's time to progress.

A good general rule of thumb for increasing weight loads is the following:

10-pound increase for lower-body exercises

5-pound increase for upper-body exercises

you also get a little more rest to recover from the heavier lifting. Remember, the key to improving your strength is to "stress" the muscle by working hard and then allow enough rest to recover to about 80 percent before the next set.

All of the variables that you see in my Newbie program work together to ensure that you get the lean, strong, feminine physique that you're after. I've worked some magic behind the scenes; all you have to do is follow my Three-Step System to Strength and you can be confident that you're on the right track! Here's a breakdown of the details of the Newbie program.

Newbie 90-Day Training Program

Workouts per week: 2

Total number of exercises: 16

Muscle Groups Worked

WORKOUT A	WORKOUT B
Legs, including Calves	Legs
Back	Chest
Biceps	Triceps
Abs	Shoulders

Program Days: 1–27 (Rest 3 full days before starting the next program segment.)

WORKOUT	EXERCISE	SETS	REPS	REST	NOTES
A	Leg Curl	2	12	:30	
	Leg Press	2	15	:30	
	Reverse Grip Pulldown	2	12	:30	
	Seated Cable Row	2	12	:30	
	Dumbbell Hammer Curl	2	12	:30	
	Calf Raise	2	15	:30	
	All Fours Crunch	2	20	:30	
	Plank on Ball	2	:20	:30	
	Total Sets:	**16**			
B	Leg Extension	2	10	:30	
	Walking Lunge	2	20	:30	Steps per leg = 40 total
	Bench Stepup	2	10	:30	Each leg
	Seated Upright Chest Fly	2	12	:30	
	Incline Dumbbell Press	2	10	:30	
	Barbell Overhead Press	2	10	:30	
	Straight Bar Cable Pressdown	2	15	:30	
	Dumbbell French Press	2	10	:30	
	Total Sets:	**16**			

Program Days: 31–57 (Rest 3 full days before starting the next program segment.)

WORKOUT	EXERCISE	SETS	REPS	REST	NOTES
A	Leg Curl	3	12	:60	
	Leg Press	3	15	:60	
	Reverse Grip Pulldown	3	12	:60	
	Seated Cable Row	2	15	:60	
	Dumbbell Hammer Curl	3	12	:60	
	Calf Raise	2	20	:60	
	All Fours Crunch	3	20	:60	
	Plank on Ball	2	:30	:60	
	Total Sets:	**21**			
B	Leg Extension	2	12	:60	
	Walking Lunge	2	24	:60	Steps per leg = 48 total
	Bench Stepup	3	10	:60	Each leg
	Seated Upright Chest Fly	2	15	:60	
	Incline Dumbbell Press	2	12	:60	
	Barbell Overhead Press	3	10	:60	
	Straight Bar Cable Pressdown	3	12	:60	
	Dumbbell French Press	2	12	:60	
	Total Sets:	**19**			

Program Days: 61–87 (Rest for 3 days after Day 87.)

WORKOUT	EXERCISE	SETS	REPS	REST	NOTES
A	Leg Curl	3	10	:75	
	Leg Press	3	12	:75	
	Reverse Grip Pulldown	3	10	:75	
	Seated Cable Row	3	12	:75	
	Dumbbell Hammer Curl	4	12	:75	
	Calf Raise	3	20	:75	
	All Fours Crunch	3	30	:75	
	Plank on Ball	3	:30	:75	
	Total Sets:	**25**			
B	Leg Extension	3	12	:75	
	Walking Lunge	3	24	:75	Steps per leg = 48 total
	Bench Stepup	3	10	:75	Each leg
	Seated Upright Chest Fly	2	12	:75	
	Incline Dumbbell Press	3	10	:75	
	Barbell Overhead Press	3	12	:75	
	Straight Bar Cable Pressdown	3	12	:75	
	Dumbbell French Press	3	15	:75	
	Total Sets:	**23**			

Q: "Am I working hard enough?"

A: Easy! Did you observe Step 2 (speed of movement) for all of your repetitions? Were the last 2 reps of your set just a wee bit sloppy? If you answered yes, you've found your sweet spot and you're definitely working hard enough! If you followed Steps 1 and 2 but your last 2 reps showed perfect technique, it's time to increase the weight.

Chapter 10
Easy Gainer

Ninety percent of women will find it difficult to increase their lean muscle mass. An "Easy Gainer" is among the lucky 10 percent with the propensity to add muscle easily. This is a blessing, not a curse. Many women who add muscle quickly tend to avoid strength training altogether if they are not interested in building mass, or if they're worried about getting too "bulky." So I've created a program that will help you to improve your strength and leanness—and boost your metabolism—without adding bulk.

Easy Gainer is your best choice if you:

> Suspect or know for certain that you add muscle easily

> Are unsure of your tendency to bulk up but know that you want to avoid it

> Want a workout that keeps you moving

> Want to improve your cardiovascular fitness during your workout

> Want a twice-weekly workout that is more challenging than the Newbie program

For years I believed that I was an Easy Gainer. But I was strength training incorrectly, and I mistook water retention for bulk. Many years later I realized that I am, without question, a Hard Gainer. If you are an experienced athlete or fitness enthusiast, you probably already know if you gain muscle easily or not. If you're not sure, don't stress about it. Anyone can use this program. However, if you're trying to decide between two programs, you'll probably have better success building lean muscle with another program.

How the Plan Works

The Easy Gainer program uses a protocol designed to create strength and body leanness without increasing muscle size. This program is the most cardiovascular of the four workouts, and it uses a lifting format called supersets. A superset consists of two different exercises that are performed back-to-back without rest in between. You do one exercise and then immediately do the second, resting only after the second exercise is completed. By limiting your rest phases, your muscles aren't able to recover fully in between sets and exercises. In addition, the pause at the point of max effort—part of Step 2 of the Three-Step System to Strength—keeps your muscles from working at full power. As a result, your body will build strength instead of increasing muscle size.

Because they limit rest periods, supersets keep your heart rate elevated more than the other three programs, allowing you to improve your cardiovascular fitness at the same time.

Easy Gainer is a full-body program divided up into two workouts per week. Each workout will take you approximately 35 to 40 minutes to complete and targets four major muscle groups. Each of the two weekly Easy Gainer workouts will include exercises for your legs, since they contain a significant amount of your body's muscle mass. (And what woman *doesn't* want to tone her legs, thighs, and butt?) You'll work your other major muscle groups only once per week. Workout A targets your legs (including calves), back, biceps, and abs. Workout B targets your legs, chest, triceps, and shoulders. In total, Easy Gainer includes 17 different exercises that work your entire body.

Your week at a glance: Because this program is quite challenging and demands strength, endurance, and cardiovascular fitness, you want to ensure adequate rest in between workouts. That's why you'll only do two workouts each week. Yes, that's more than enough to see results! The ideal split allows 2 days of rest in between Workouts A and B.

Here are a few ways you could organize your workout schedule.

Monday: Workout A
Thursday: Workout B

or

Wednesday: Workout A
Saturday: Workout B

or

Tuesday: Workout A
Friday: Workout B

The month-by-month progression:

Month 1: Your workout will include four supersets, or eight total exercises, except for Workout A, which also includes two sets of Calf Raises as a sort of stand-alone superset. Each superset (except for the one that works your calves) includes two different exercises for two different body parts. You'll perform the two exercises in order with no rest between the two sets. You'll rest for 30 seconds after the second exercise and then repeat the superset.

Months 2 and 3: You'll increase the number of sets and reps overall each month and decrease the rest phase. By the 3rd month you'll be rocking out a big workout (and burning major calories!) in just 40 minutes!

Easy Gainer Quick Look

Right for you if: You know or suspect that you have a propensity to build muscle easily.

Workouts per week: 2
Full body: Yes!
Skill level: Beginner to Intermediate
Number of exercises: 17
Time per workout: 35–40 minutes

Easy Gainer 90-Day Training Program

Workouts per week: 2

Total number of exercises: 17

Muscle Groups Worked

WORKOUT A	WORKOUT B
Legs, including Calves	Legs
Back	Chest
Biceps	Triceps
Abs	Shoulders

Program Days: 1–27 (Rest 3 full days before starting the next program segment.)

WORKOUT		EXERCISE	SETS	REPS	REST	NOTES
A	**Superset 1**	Leg Press	2	12	0	
		Reverse Grip Pulldown	2	15	0	
					:30	Rest between supersets
	Superset 2	Walking Lunge	2	24	0	Stepping forward with each leg = 1 rep
		Bent–Over Barbell Row	2	15	0	
					:30	Rest between supersets
	Superset 3	Dumbbell Hammer Curl	2	15	0	
		All Fours Crunch	2	20	0	
					:30	Rest between supersets
	Superset 4	Alternating Dumbbell Supinated Curl	2	15	0	Curling each arm = 1 rep
		Bicycle	2	30	0	A complete cycle of each leg = 1 rep
					:30	Rest between supersets
		Calf Raise	2	15		Perform as a superset
	Total Sets:		**18**			

WORKOUT		EXERCISE	SETS	REPS	REST	NOTES
B	**Superset 1**	Bench Stepup	2	12	0	Complete all reps on one leg before switching to the next leg.
		Incline Dumbbell Press	2	15	0	
					:30	Rest between supersets
	Superset 2	Leg Curl	2	12	0	
		Flat Dumbbell Fly	2	12	0	
					:30	Rest between supersets
	Superset 3	Dumbbell Upright Row	2	15	0	
		Dumbbell French Press	2	15	0	
					:30	Rest between supersets
	Superset 4	Dumbbell Bent Arm Side Raise	2	12	0	
		Overhead Rope Extension	2	15	0	
					:30	Rest between supersets
	Total Sets:		**16**			

Program Days: 31–57 (Rest 3 full days before starting the next program segment.)

WORKOUT		EXERCISE	SETS	REPS	REST	NOTES
A	Superset 1	Leg Press	3	15	0	
		Reverse Grip Pulldown	3	15	0	
					:15	Rest between supersets
	Superset 2	Walking Lunge	2	30	0	Steps per leg = 60 total
		Bent–Over Barbell Row	2	15		
					:15	Rest between supersets
	Superset 3	Dumbbell Hammer Curl	2	20	0	
		All Fours Crunch	2	30	0	
					:15	Rest between supersets
	Superset 4	Alternating Dumbbell Supinated Curl	2	15	0	Per arm = 30 total
		Bicycle	2	40	0	Per leg = 80 total
					:15	Rest between supersets
		Calf Raise	2	15		Perform as a straight set
	Total Sets:		**20**			

WORKOUT		EXERCISE	SETS	REPS	REST	NOTES
B	Superset 1	Bench Stepup	3	12	0	Each leg
		Incline Dumbbell Press	3	15	0	
					:15	Rest between supersets
	Superset 2	Leg Curl	2	15	0	
		Flat Dumbbell Fly	2	15	0	
					:15	Rest between supersets
	Superset 3	Dumbbell Upright Row	2	15	0	
		Dumbbell French Press	2	15	0	
					:15	Rest between supersets
	Superset 4	Dumbbell Bent Arm Side Raise	2	15	0	
		Overhead Rope Extension	2	20	0	
					:15	Rest between supersets
	Total Sets:		**18**			

Program Days: 61–87

WORKOUT		EXERCISE	SETS	REPS	REST	NOTES
A		Leg Press	3	20	0	
	Superset 1	Reverse Grip Pulldown	3	15	0	
					0	Rest between supersets
		Walking Lunge	2	40	0	Steps per leg = 80 total
	Superset 2	Bent–Over Barbell Row	2	20	0	
		Dumbbell Hammer Curl	3	15	0	
	Superset 3	All Fours Crunch	3	30	0	
		Alternating Dumbbell Supinated Curl	3	15	0	Per arm = 30 total
	Superset 4	Bicycle	3	50	0	Per leg = 100 total
		Calf Raise	2	15	0	Perform as a straight set
	Total Sets:		**24**			

WORKOUT		EXERCISE	SETS	REPS	REST	NOTES
B		Bench Stepup	3	15	0	Each leg
	Superset 1	Incline Dumbbell Press	3	15	0	
		Leg Curl	3	15	0	
	Superset 2	Flat Dumbbell Fly	3	15	0	
		Dumbbell Upright Row	2	15	0	
	Superset 3	Dumbbell French Press	2	20	0	
		Dumbbell Bent Arm Side Raise	3	15	0	
	Superset 4	Overhead Rope Extension	3	20	0	
	Total Sets:		**22**			

Chapter 11
Hard Gainer

A "Hard Gainer" is someone whose physiology makes it tough to build muscle mass. Is that you? Probably. Because of our hormones, most women fall into this category. It is just very hard for us to increase muscle size and strength, period. We have to work just a bit harder than other folks in order to create that fit, sexy physique that we want. Ninety percent of my clients and women with whom I consult are true Hard Gainers. And in order to inspire change, this group needs a very specific workout program.

The inspiration for this plan comes from thousands of conversations with women about what they truly want. Most of the time, that's something more than just a smaller version of their current bodies. If you are ready to discover a new kind of strength, to truly redesign your body, and to fire up your metabolism, this program is made just for you.

This program works best if you have at least 6 months of experience in strength training. That being said, if you are brand new to strength training and know you can recover from workouts very efficiently without a lot of soreness, even after intense exercise, you could follow this program.

Hard Gainer is right for you if you:

> Want to take your fitness to the next level
> Want the strong look that comes with increasing your lean muscle mass

> Are eager to discover a new kind of inner strength

> Want to supercharge your metabolism in order to burn body fat all day long

> Want to create true and lasting stamina

> Want to improve your body mechanics and reduce aches and pains

> Feel invigorated by hard workouts

> Are ready, once and for all, to achieve the body of your dreams

How the Plan Works

Hard Gainer includes 3 days of strength training, compared to just 2 in the Newbie and Easy Gainer plans. By breaking this full-body program into more frequent workouts, you're able to spend more time on each body part, ensuring that you get the stimulus you really need to see a dramatic change.

On this program, you'll work very hard during every set and then take longer rest periods between sets. During the last few reps of each exercise, you'll be working at close to 90 percent of your ability, so a longer rest phase allows you to recover before the next set. The name of the game here is work hard, rest hard. This program is designed to expose you to extremes. Each of the three weekly workouts will take you approximately 35 to 45 minutes and targets three major muscle groups. Because there are more workouts in the week, you're able to put more love into key muscle groups, like legs and abs—two areas that my female clients always want to firm up.

> Workout A focuses on legs, back, and abs.

> Workout B targets shoulders, biceps, triceps, and calves.

> Workout C works legs again, chest, and more abs.

Your week at a glance: As with all strength-training programs, it's important to allow for rest in between workouts. Because there are 3 days of workouts in this program, you'll schedule 1 day of rest between sessions, unless you choose to exercise on weekends. You have a few options for your weekly schedule.

**Hard Gainer
Quick Look**

Right for you if:
You want to make
over your metabo-
lism and get a
toned, athletic look.

**Workouts per
week:** 3
Full body: Yes!
Skill level:
Advanced-
Beginner to
Advanced-
Intermediate
**Number of
exercises:** 19
Time per workout:
35–45 minutes

Monday: Workout A
Wednesday: Workout B
Friday: Workout C

or

Monday: Workout A
Wednesday: Workout B
Saturday: Workout C

or

Monday: Workout A
Thursday: Workout B
Saturday: Workout C

The month-by-month progression: The 1st month of this program you'll be completing two sets of all the exercises with a high number of reps per set and moderate rest. By the 3rd month, you'll be adding sets but doing fewer reps per set with heavier weights and taking longer rests. The extra rest allows your muscles to recover a bit more so that you can work harder during the sets. Again, the Last 2 Reps Rule will help you determine the proper weight to use as you increase the load.

Q: "Am I working too hard?"

A: Chances are if you follow my Three-Step System to Strength on any of the 90-day training plans, you will be working at the right effort level. If you feel that you are straining or overexerting in any way, simply scale back your effort. If you feel totally wrecked after your workouts and have chronic muscle soreness, take it easy for 1 to 2 weeks. This will give your body time to fully recover.

Hard Gainer 90-Day Training Program

Workouts per week: 3
Total number of exercises: 19

Muscle Groups Worked

WORKOUT A	WORKOUT B	WORKOUT C
Legs	Shoulders	Legs
Back	Biceps	Chest
Abs	Triceps	Abs
	Calves	

Program Days: 1–27 (Rest 3 full days before starting the next program segment.)

WORKOUT	EXERCISE	SETS	REPS	REST	NOTES
A	Leg Curl	2	12	:60	
	Leg Press	2	15	:60	
	Reverse Grip Pulldown	2	15	:60	
	Bent–Over Barbell Row	2	15	:60	
	All Fours Crunch	2	20	:60	
	Bicycle	2	30	:60	Per leg = 60 total
	Total Sets:	**12**			
B	Barbell Overhead Press	2	15	:60	
	Dumbbell Bent Arm Side Raise	2	12	:60	
	Straight Bar Cable Pressdown	2	15	:60	
	Dumbbell French Press	2	12	:60	
	Straight Bar Cable Curl	2	12	:60	
	Calf Raise	2	20	:60	
	Total Sets:	**12**			
C	Goblet Squat	2	15	:60	
	Walking Lunge	2	24	:60	Steps per leg = 48 total
	Leg Extension	2	15	:60	
	Flat Bench Press	2	12	:60	
	Flat Dumbbell Fly	2	12	:60	
	Hanging Knee-Up	2	10	:60	
	Weighted Ball Flexion	2	20	:60	
	Total Sets:	**14**			

Program Days: 31–57 (Rest 3 full days before starting the next program segment.)

WORKOUT	EXERCISE	SETS	REPS	REST	NOTES
A	Leg Curl	2	12	:75	
	Leg Press	3	12	:75	
	Reverse Grip Pulldown	3	12	:75	
	Bent–Over Barbell Row	2	12	:75	
	All Fours Crunch	2	25	:75	
	Bicycle	2	50	:75	Per leg = 100 total
	Total Sets:	**14**			
B	Barbell Overhead Press	3	12	:75	
	Dumbbell Bent Arm Side Raise	2	12	:75	
	Straight Bar Cable Pressdown	3	12	:75	
	Dumbbell French Press	2	12	:75	
	Straight Bar Cable Curl	3	12	:75	
	Calf Raise	2	18	:75	
	Total Sets:	**15**			
C	Goblet Squat	3	12	:75	
	Walking Lunge	2	24	:75	Steps per leg = 48 total
	Leg Extension	2	12	:75	
	Flat Bench Press	2	12	:75	
	Flat Dumbbell Fly	3	12	:75	
	Hanging Knee-Up	2	15	:75	
	Weighted Ball Flexion	3	20	:75	
	Total Sets:	**17**			

Program Days: 61–87

WORKOUT	EXERCISE	SETS	REPS	REST	NOTES
A	Leg Curl	3	10	:90	
	Leg Press	3	10	:90	
	Reverse Grip Pulldown	3	10	:90	
	Bent–Over Barbell Row	3	12	:90	
	All Fours Crunch	3	30	:90	
	Bicycle	2	70	:90	Per leg = 140 total
	Total Sets:	**17**			
B	Barbell Overhead Press	3	10	:90	
	Dumbbell Bent Arm Side Raise	3	10	:90	
	Straight Bar Cable Pressdown	3	12	:90	
	Dumbbell French Press	3	12	:90	
	Straight Bar Cable Curl	3	10	:90	
	Calf Raise	3	15	:90	
	Total Sets:	**18**			
C	Goblet Squat	3	10	:90	
	Walking Lunge	3	20	:90	Steps per leg = 40 total
	Leg Extension	3	12	:90	
	Flat Bench Press	3	10	:90	
	Flat Dumbbell Fly	3	10	:90	
	Hanging Knee-Up	3	15	:90	
	Weighted Ball Flexion	3	20	:90	
	Total Sets:	**21**			

What Hard Gainers Must Do Every Workout

Technique is always important—but it's especially crucial if you're following the Hard Gainer program. Because you're going to be lifting heavier weights, your body is going to want to go on autopilot, using your strongest and most dominant muscles to perform the movement. The problem is, those aren't always the muscles you want to be working. Sloppy technique during this plan will temper your results. At worst, it'll set you up for injuries down the line. You must be extra careful to perform the exercises using perfect technique as your loads increase. So repeat after me: Technique trumps all!

Chapter 12
Radical Transformation

Do you work out—or do you train?

There will come a time in your weight-lifting journey when you will wake up one day and feel something new. You will find yourself with a solid, unshakable sense of resolve about your fitness life. This will be the day when you graduate. You will no longer call your visit to the gym a "workout"; instead, you will call it a "training session." This is the moment when you no longer view your workouts as lifting weights. It is the day when you have begun strength training.

When that day arrives, you will be ready for the Radical Transformation plan, a higher-volume program intended to take you from an intermediate level to an advanced level. This is the program that took me from fit to an undeniable example of superfit. It is the program that caused my personal shift from committed to passionate.

This program is for you if you have been consistently strength training for at least 6 months and are ready to take your fitness to the next level. One goal of Radical Transformation is to significantly increase your lean muscle mass while decreasing your body fat to an athletic range of between 17 and 20 percent.

If you are new to strength training, it is essential that you first begin with one of the other 90-day plans and graduate to this one. It may be tempting to dive into the deep end, but you will ultimately see better results if you build a strong strength foundation first.

Radical Transformation is right for you if you:

> Have been strength training consistently for at least 6 months
> Are ready to take your fitness to a level your body has never experienced before
> Are interested in adding lean muscle mass
> Want to cultivate a deeper sense of inner strength
> Are dedicated to your time at the gym and eager to challenge your body's limits

Crush It!

Following this program will force you to dig deep and challenge yourself in a very new, very significant way. There will be moments during this program when you will see a clear distinction between comfortable and uncomfortable. There will be moments when you will want to quit and be faced with the decision of overcoming the challenge. In order to change your body in a radical way, you must push it beyond its current comfort zone. Each and every set should prompt you to make a concerted decision to fight, to overcome, and to grow.

How the Plan Works

Radical Transformation is a full-body program split into four workouts per week. Each workout will take you approximately 60 minutes to complete and targets two or three muscle groups. The 4-day split includes 30 different exercises and is broken down like this:

Workout A: Upper legs and lower legs
Workout B: Back and abs

Workout C: Legs, chest, and abs

Workout D: Shoulders, biceps, and triceps

Your week at a glance: Because the emphasis is on harder, more intense workouts, it is best to space out the four weekly sessions as much as possible. There will be two workouts that occur on consecutive days, and it's best to put a day of rest in between the other workouts. In other words, try to avoid training 3 days in a row. Here are two good options.

Monday: Workout A
Tuesday: Workout B
Thursday: Workout C
Saturday: Workout D

or

Tuesday: Workout A
Thursday: Workout B
Saturday: Workout C
Sunday: Workout D

The month-by-month progression: Decades of research show that the most effective way to improve strength is through a program that emphasizes heavier loads with longer rest phases between sets. So the name of the game here is to lift heavy and work hard during each set so that you need a longer break. The goal of the rest phase is to allow your muscles to recover to between 70 and 80 percent so that you can enter the next set saying, "All right, let's *do* this!"

Dividing this program up into four different workouts allows for more time dedicated to each muscle group. You'll be performing more sets, more reps, and longer rest phases over the course of the 90 days. In the 3rd month you will be performing up to 34 total sets in one workout. This high number of sets puts a high demand on your muscles and is a proven method for inspiring change.

Radical Transforma-tion Quick Look

Right for you if: You are ready to take your body to the next level and inspire significant changes in your body fat and lean muscle mass. You have a solid strength-training background and are ready to commit to an ambitious plan.

Workouts per week: 4
Full body: Yes!
Skill level: Intermediate to Advanced-Intermediate
Number of exercises: 30
Time per workout: 60–70 minutes

Radical Transformation 90-Day Training Program

Workouts per week: 4
Total number of exercises: 30

Muscle Groups Worked

WORKOUT A	WORKOUT B	WORKOUT C	WORKOUT D
Legs	Back	Legs	Shoulders
Calves	Abs	Chest	Biceps
		Abs	Triceps

Program Days: 1–27 (Rest 3 full days before starting the next program segment.)

WORKOUT	EXERCISE	SETS	REPS	REST	NOTES
A	Leg Curl	3	15/12/10	:90	Increase weight each set.
	Goblet Squat	3	15/12/10	:90	Increase weight each set.
	Walking Lunge	2	30/24	:90	Steps per leg = 60/48 total
	Leg Press	2	12/12	:90	
	Calf Raise	3	20/18/15	:90	
	Total Sets:	**13**			
B	Reverse Grip Pulldown	3	15/12/10	:90	Increase weight each set.
	Seated Cable Row	2	12/12	:90	Increase weight each set.
	Assisted Pullup	2	12/12	:90	Increase weight each set.
	Lying Dumbbell Pullover	2	15/12	:90	Increase weight each set.
	Hanging Knee-Up	1	20	:90	
	Weighted Ball Flexion	2	30/30	:90	
	Bicycle	1	80	:90	Per leg = 160 total
	Total Sets:	**13**			

WORKOUT	EXERCISE	SETS	REPS	REST	NOTES
C	Bench Stepup	2	12/12	:90	Complete all reps with one leg before exercising the other leg. Increase weight each set.
	Leg Press	3	15/15/15	:90	Increase weight each set.
	Deadlift	2	15/12	:90	Increase weight each set.
	Leg Extension	2	15/15	:90	Increase weight each set.
	Seated Upright Chest Fly	2	15/12	:90	Increase weight each set.
	Flat Bench Press	2	15/12	:90	Increase weight each set.
	Incline Dumbbell Press	2	15/12	:90	Increase weight each set.
	Plank on Ball	1	:60	:90	Increase weight each set.
	All Fours Crunch	2	40/35	:90	Increase weight each set.
	Weighted Ball Flexion	2	20/20	:90	Increase weight each set.
	Total Sets:	**20**			
D	Barbell Overhead Press	3	15/12/10	:90	Increase weight each set.
	Dumbbell Upright Row	2	12/12	:90	Increase weight each set.
	Dumbbell Bent Arm Side Raise	2	12/12	:90	Increase weight each set.
	Reverse Dumbbell Fly	3	12/12/10	:90	Increase weight each set.
	Straight Bar Cable Pressdown	2	18/15	:90	Increase weight each set.
	Overhead Rope Extension	2	15/12	:90	Increase weight each set.
	Dumbbell French Press	2	15/12	:90	Increase weight each set.
	Straight Bar Cable Curl	3	12/12/12	:90	Increase weight each set.
	Dumbbell Hammer Curl	2	15/12	:90	Increase weight each set.
	Total Sets:	**21**			

Program Days: 31–57 (Rest 3 full days before starting the next program segment.)

WORKOUT	EXERCISE	SETS	REPS	REST	NOTES
A	Leg Curl	3	15/12/10	:75	Increase weight each set.
	Goblet Squat	3	15/12/10	:75	Increase weight each set.
	Walking Lunge	3	30/24/20	:75	Steps per leg = 60/48/40 total
	Leg Press	3	12/12/10	:75	
	Calf Raise	4	20/18/15/15	:75	
	Total Sets:	**16**			
B	Reverse Grip Pulldown	4	15/12/10/10	:75	Increase weight each set.
	Seated Cable Row	3	12/12/10	:75	Increase weight each set.
	Assisted Pullup	3	12/12/10	:75	Increase weight each set.
	Lying Dumbbell Pullover	3	15/12/12	:75	Increase weight each set.
	Hanging Knee-Up	2	20/20	:75	Increase weight each set.
	Weighted Ball Flexion	3	30/30/30	:75	Increase weight each set.
	Bicycle	2	80/80	:75	Per leg = 160 total
	Total Sets:	**20**			
C	Bench Stepup	2	12/12	:75	Increase weight each set.
	Leg Press	4	15/15/12/12	:75	Increase weight each set.
	Deadlift	3	15/12/12	:75	Increase weight each set.
	Leg Extension	2	15/15	:75	Increase weight each set.
	Seated Upright Chest Fly	3	15/12/12	:75	Increase weight each set.
	Flat Bench Press	2	15/12	:75	Increase weight each set.
	Incline Dumbbell Press	3	15/12/12	:75	Increase weight each set.
	Plank on Ball	2	:60	:75	Increase weight each set.
	All Fours Crunch	3	40/35/30	:75	Increase weight each set.
	Weighted Ball Flexion	2	20/20	:75	Increase weight each set.
	Total Sets:	**26**			

WORKOUT	EXERCISE	SETS	REPS	REST	NOTES
D	Barbell Overhead Press	3	15/12/10	:75	Increase weight each set.
	Dumbbell Upright Row	3	12/12/10	:75	Increase weight each set.
	Dumbbell Bent Arm Side Raise	3	12/12/10	:75	Increase weight each set.
	Reverse Dumbbell Fly	3	12/12/10	:75	Increase weight each set.
	Straight Bar Cable Pressdown	3	18/15/12	:75	Increase weight each set.
	Overhead Rope Extension	3	15/12/12	:75	Increase weight each set.
	Dumbbell French Press	3	15/12/10	:75	Increase weight each set.
	Straight Bar Cable Curl	3	12/12/10	:75	Increase weight each set.
	Dumbbell Hammer Curl	3	15/12/10	:75	Increase weight each set.
	Total Sets:	**27**			

Program Days: 61–87

WORKOUT	EXERCISE	SETS	REPS	REST	NOTES
A	Leg Curl	4	15/12/10/10	:60	Increase weight each set.
	Goblet Squat	4	15/12/10/10	:60	Increase weight each set.
	Walking Lunge	3	30/24/20	:60	Steps per leg = 60/48/40 total
	Leg Press	4	12/12/10/10	:60	
	Calf Raise	5	20/18/15/15/15	:60	
	Total Sets:	**20**		:60	
B	Reverse Grip Pulldown	4	15/12/10/10	:60	Increase weight each set.
	Seated Cable Row	4	15/12/10/10	:60	Increase weight each set.
	Assisted Pullup	4	12/12/10/10	:60	Increase weight each set.
	Lying Dumbbell Pullover	3	15/12/12	:60	Increase weight each set.
	Hanging Knee-Up	3	20/20/20	:60	Increase weight each set.
	Weighted Ball Flexion	3	30/30/30	:60	Increase weight each set.
	Bicycle	2	80/80	:60	Per leg = 160 total
	Total Sets:	**23**			

(continued)

WORKOUT	EXERCISE	SETS	REPS	REST	NOTES
C	Bench Stepup	3	12/12/10	:60	Increase weight each set.
	Leg Press	4	15/15/12/12	:60	
	Deadlift	4	15/12/12/10	:60	
	Leg Extension	3	15/15/12	:60	
	Seated Upright Chest Fly	3	15/12/12	:60	
	Flat Bench Press	3	15/12/10	:60	
	Incline Dumbbell Press	4	15/12/12/10	:60	
	Plank on Ball	3	:60	:60	
	All Fours Crunch	4	40/35/30/25	:60	
	Weighted Ball Flexion	3	20/20/20	:60	
	Total Sets:	**34**			
D	Barbell Overhead Press	4	15/12/10/10	:60	Increase weight each set.
	Dumbbell Upright Row	4	12/12/10/10	:60	
	Dumbbell Bent Arm Side Raise	3	12/12/10	:60	
	Reverse Dumbbell Fly	4	12/12/10/10	:60	
	Straight Bar Cable Pressdown	4	18/15/12/12	:60	
	Overhead Rope Extension	3	15/12/12	:60	
	Dumbbell French Press	3	15/12/10	:60	
	Straight Bar Cable Curl	4	12/12/10/10	:60	
	Dumbbell Hammer Curl	4	15/12/10/10	:60	
	Total Sets:	**33**			

The Most Confusing Gym Riddle—Answered

Pretty much every piece of equipment in the gym is different in terms of how you'll experience its weight loads. For example, you might have two different leg press machines in your gym that look very similar. One might be a plate-loaded machine and the other pin loaded. First, you need to understand the difference: Plate-loaded equipment uses round weight plates that range from 5 to 45 pounds, while pin-loaded equipment has a vertical weight stack and a pin that allows you to select the desired weight; it usually increases by 5 to 15 pounds per pinhole.

Your ability on each machine could be very different in terms of the amount of weight used. For example, you might be able to perform your sets at 50 pounds on the pin-loaded machine and 90 pounds on the plate-loaded one. So what's going on? Are you really that much stronger today?

Not quite. Each piece of equipment has its own system of weight gradation, and the ultimate goal for you is to increase your ability on each piece of equipment. All you have to do is come back to my Three-Step System to Strength in order to find your sweet spot. By observing my three steps, you will be able to figure out the perfect effort level for your body in any gym, with any equipment. Think of the weight load on any machine as simply an "effort level" rather than an absolute number.

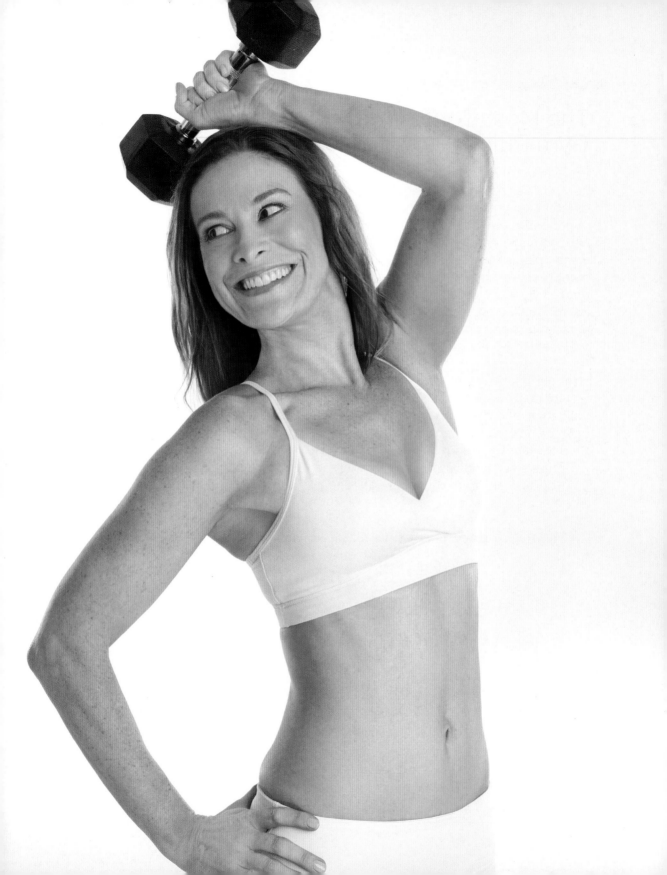

Part IV
Everything Else You Need to Know

Lift
to Get
Lean

Chapter 13
Questions, Answers, and Tips for Your First Workout

Depending on your gym, the weight room can be an intimidating place at first glance. All those weird machines and industrial-looking hunks of iron. All those people who look like they know what they're doing clanking heavy weights. All those men!

You're probably thinking, "*Sheesh*. What did I get myself into?" Relax. You paid your dues just like everyone else, so you have a right to be there, too. Besides, you'll find that, for the most part, folks at the gym are pretty nice and often very helpful.

Just like outside in the real world, there are social skills and simple rules of etiquette at the gym that help everyone play nice in the same sandbox. In this chapter, I'll review some of those commonsense rules so you feel comfortable and confident. I'll give you useful hints and tips to make your first workout a lot of fun, and I'll tackle some frequently asked questions like those starting on the next page.

What's the best time of day to work out?

The short answer is, the time of day when you'll do it!

After years of personal trial and error, client observation, and research review, I've come to the conclusion that the best time of day to work out is:

1. When you are most likely to do it
2. When your energy is at its best, or simply
3. When you *feel* like doing it

Research suggests that there are some hormonal benefits to working out in the morning, when your natural cortisol levels are high. Indeed, I have clients who are morning people and have great energy at 5:00 a.m. Others will growl at me if I suggest a 7:00 a.m. appointment. The time of day that you work out is truly a personal preference. The most important thing is that you stay consistent and show up for your workouts. If you prefer to exercise when the gym is relatively empty, avoid the peak hours, such as before and after work; 11:00 a.m. or 3:00 p.m. might be perfect for you if you have a flexible work schedule. The point is, schedule your workouts at times when you are most likely to succeed.

Should I warm up before lifting?

The phrase "warm up" has always made me giggle a bit. The last time I checked, most humans are walking around at about 98.6°F. That seems pretty warm to me! The purpose of a so-called warmup isn't to actually warm your body but rather to *prepare your body metabolically* for your workout. The idea is to shift your body from stationary, at-rest mode to movement mode. You want to rev up your metabolism and energy production for your training session. And the best way to do that is with 6 to 10 minutes of cardio activity, such as stationary cycling, running on a treadmill, using a rowing machine or elliptical, or doing old-school calisthenics.

Start out slowly, then increase intensity. For example, if you choose to warm up on the treadmill, begin with a comfortable walk. Then, over the course of the warmup, increase the speed or incline so that you end a bit sweaty and energized. You don't want the warmup to cause fatigue; you want it to energize you.

Is there any special equipment I should bring to the gym?

I never leave for a workout without the following four essentials.

1. *My own music.* Research shows that listening to music during workouts improves mood, decreases perceived discomfort, and fosters better energy. But I may not like the tunes playing on the gym loudspeakers, so I always bring my favorite workout playlist on my phone.

2. *A sports watch.* A watch on your wrist with a timer function is really helpful for timing the rest phases of your training program. You may want a sports watch that has a heart rate monitor, too, but outside of that, you don't need a watch that is super fancy. I have a very basic sports watch from New Balance that I have used day in and day out for 6 years. It's simple and works perfectly for my needs. You might have to do a little research to find one that is simple. It seems that bells and whistles are the rage these days and many sports watches have frills that translate into a higher price tag. All you need is something that says "Start" and "Stop." And this should run you less than $45.

3. *Proper footwear.* Avoid wearing running shoes. Many have a heel-to-toe drop of more than 8 millimeters; some are as high as 12. That's like wearing high heels! You want to wear training shoes that keep your feet flat and your heels close to the ground. This improves stability of your ankles and will force greater activation of your hamstrings and glutes during leg exercises. Do some research to find a flexible, comfortable training shoe. Otherwise, a flat running shoe is your second-best bet. Just make sure that you buy one with a low heel-to-toe drop. I prefer a training shoe that is between 0 and 8 millimeters.

4. *A workout log.* In the appendix, you'll find a simple system to jot down notes during your workout. Keep track of your reps and sets and weight amounts. A visual reminder of your progress

can be very motivating. Take notes about how you feel—for example, "I feel tired today" or "Great energy"—to give your performance a frame of reference.

What should I eat before a workout?

You are a Ferrari. You need high-octane fuel in order to zoom. So fueling your body the right way before a workout is something to take seriously. You do want to eat something, but not too much. If you fill up before a workout, your digestive system will kick into high gear, stealing blood away from your muscles at just the time when your muscles need blood to perform optimally. To keep this from happening *and* provide your body with enough fuel to power your workout, you have two options: Eat a full, balanced meal about 2 hours before your workout, or have a small meal (call it a snack) of 150 to 300 calories a half hour to an hour before you hit the weights. That'll keep your blood sugar stable and provide enough energy for your muscles to work with. What to eat? Have a mix of protein and easy-to-digest carbohydrates with very little fat. Fruit paired with string cheese or a hard-cooked egg with some grapes are good choices, but my favorite preworkout fuel options are half of a protein bar; a smoothie made with whey protein powder, water, berries, and flax oil; or low-fat Greek yogurt with agave nectar.

Eating after your workout is important, too; it provides fuel for muscle repair and recovery. You'll want to have something within 30 minutes of the end of your workout, the time when your body needs to replenish glycogen (muscle fuel) spent during your workout. So, again, have a mix of carbohydrates and protein. The snack should contain about 20 grams of protein, the building block of muscle tissue. That's why a protein shake is an ideal postworkout mini meal. It's easy to consume and provides a jolt of protein. The best postworkout protein shake appears to be one that contains a blend of soy, whey, and casein proteins, according to a study in the *Journal of Nutrition*. A test panel of exercisers was given either a protein drink containing all three types of powdered protein or a drink made with only whey protein, and then researchers measured how quickly the participants' bodies broke down the proteins into amino acids used to build new muscle. It turned out that the protein shakes containing soy, whey, and casein generated longer-lasting protein synthesis, providing a better cocktail for muscle repair and growth.

Finally, be sure to drink plenty of water before, during, and after your workout, but especially before, when most people don't think to hydrate. So drink 16 to 20 ounces of cool water 2 hours prior to your workout.

What should I wear to work out?

Don't be afraid to show off your shape. Besides, there are practical reasons to wear form-fitting workout clothes. Loose, floppy sweats can restrict your movement. What's worse, they can get caught in an exercise machine or make you trip. Your clothing doesn't have to be spandex-tight, but shorts, tops, or bottoms that hug your body make it easier to see your muscles working. That's good for checking your form and also for motivating yourself. When you see how firm your muscles look, you'll be more inclined to push yourself harder. And it feels great to believe that you look nice. Social science studies have shown that people feel more confident and perform better when they take pride in their appearance and dress nicely for special occasions. I think transforming your body is a very special occasion! I want you to be focused on how much you're enjoying your workout and not on a wardrobe malfunction. Whatever makes you feel comfortable is the best bet.

Here are some spectacular workout clothes to consider.

Training shoes. The foundation that you put under your body is so important for setting up proper alignment. Wearing a shoe that is designed for your activities will optimize everything that you do in the gym. Also, footwear is the only thing between your body and the unforgiving ground. Your body needs good support to prevent unnecessary wear and tear on your muscles, joints, and tendons. Be sure to choose a cross-training or training shoe that is comfortable but also supportive. The shoe should be flexible enough to allow natural movement for the exercises that require ankle and foot flexion. Also, try to choose a shoe with a low heel-to-toe drop. This means that your heel will sit closer to the floor (unlike with a running shoe) and will allow you to better engage the muscles of your lower body and core. I am a big fan of anything that New Balance creates for their women's training shoes. I am particularly fond of the Minimus training shoe.

Fitted leggings or capris. I tend to default to fitted leggings and capris for my workouts. I like the coverage and sense of support. The most important factors in choosing good workout pants are comfort, coverage, and breathability. You want to feel totally unrestricted in all of your movements. There's nothing worse than feeling limited during a Deadlift or Walking Lunge! I always check the fit and comfort of the waistband, then do a few movements to make sure the pants stretch everywhere I need them to! Stretch fabrics can sometimes cause a transparency in the fabric. Be sure to give your pants a full stretch and check to make sure they stay opaque throughout all of your exercises. You can check this by sitting down into a crouched position and looking at your knees to see if any skin shows through the material. Finally, you want to make sure the fabric is a tech fabric designed to wick moisture and breathe. New Balance has a line of premium pants for women called Psyche that I really love.

Sports bra. There is nothing worse than an ill-fitting sports bra that chafes, and there is nothing better than a sports bra that works as it should! I remember in the early '90s, when there was absolutely no technology for women's athletic apparel. I would wear three sports bras in order to get enough support. All that material created chafing. It was miserable. Thankfully, there are so many awesome brands providing options for women based on size, style preferences, and activities. This is an area where it's worth spending a little extra money to get one that is right for you. Your sports bra should be so comfortable and supportive that you forget you're wearing one. Shop around and try out different styles. Consider what style you prefer aesthetically and any activities where you will be jumping up and down. Be sure to test a few options to find one or two that are perfect for you.

Tops. Gone are the days of oversized, leftover cotton college T-shirts. Save those for the weekend! You really want fitted tops of tech fabrics made for wicking and moisture control. If you prefer Ts over tank tops, choose fitted styles. Remember the section on using mirrors during your workouts? It's important to use mirrors to watch your technique during exercises. Fitted tops make assessing technique much more accurate. There are so many great options for all budgets. Consider looking online for last season's styles that are on sale!

What's the protocol for using the equipment in a busy gym, and how do I ask to use a machine or barbell?

Good question. Calling dibs on a piece of equipment can be touchy, but it's essential sometimes. Some workouts in this book require you to perform multiple sets on one piece of equipment with a short rest phase in between each set. In order to complete all of your sets, you may end up using a piece of equipment for 6 to 8 minutes straight. And that may feel like a long time if your gym is busy and someone else is interested in using the equipment. I believe that if you are the first to grab a machine or piece of equipment, you have every right to spend as much time as you need for your workout. To some degree, you should feel perfectly comfortable taking your time and sitting on the machine during your rest phases. Some days I want to stay very tight to my rest phases and don't want to be interrupted during my workout. On these days, I stay on my machine during rest phases to send the signal that I intend to perform another set and that I'm not open to sharing the machine. While this behavior is perfectly legit, it can make others a bit unhappy. We are social creatures after all, and eventually someone waiting to use the machine you are on is going to get pissy with you. Therefore, it's more socially graceful to be aware of others sniffing out your machine or barbell and to say something. Just explain, "I'm doing back-to-back sets and I have X more to go." They'll get it and appreciate you giving them a time frame. It's all about courtesy. Alternatively, if you notice that someone wants to use your machine, it's always nice to offer to let that person "work in with you." This means you will take turns using the machine. You'll rest while she is working and vice versa.

On some occasions, you'll be the one wondering who's using the equipment. Pause for a moment and look around before taking over a machine to make sure someone isn't just on a rest break. If someone is still using the machine, that person will be nearby keeping an eye on it and will run over to tell you when you approach the equipment. A good way to annoy gym regulars is by taking over equipment they were using. But again, it's a simple gesture to take a moment to look around and make sure that a piece of equipment is not being used and if it is to just ask if you could "work in." At the end of the day, you'll enjoy your gym visits more if you play nice with others. You'll do fine if you remember to use common courtesy.

Speaking of courtesy, here's another sticky situation to be aware of: leaving your sweat on a bench or machine. You'll be sure to make more friends at the gym if you clean up your sweat when you're finished with a piece of equipment. On top of being hygienic, a towel also makes exercise equipment more comfy as it provides a barrier between your skin and the sticky vinyl covering on most machines.

How do I get over feeling so awkward among so many men in the weight room?

When I ask women what keeps them from exploring the weights section at the gym, I usually get two answers.

1. I don't know how to use the equipment.
2. I feel out of place in a gym full of guys.

So, it helps to know that most women feel a little intimidated by the scene. Guys aren't used to seeing women in the gym, after all. Therefore, they might be staring at you because (a) you're pretty or (b) they think they are seeing an alien. They just aren't used to us being there!

I remember a day about 8 years ago when I was still getting comfortable—truly comfortable—in the free-weights section of a local Gold's Gym. I had just finished a set on the bench press and was sitting on it during my rest phase. If you're not familiar with this piece of equipment, it uses a standard-size Olympic bar that weighs 45 pounds unloaded. At that time in my strength-training journey, I could only lift the weight of the bar. As I was resting before my next set, a man came up and snarled: "Can I get in there?"

Interpretation: "I want to use the bench press and you are in my way."

Being the hot-tempered redhead that I am, I stood up and said, "No! I'm still working!" not in my nicest voice. He stammered a bit and then said, "But you're not even using any weight!" as though I was wasting my time on that exercise. Oh boy, I got mad: "Are you blind? I'm a *female*! Forty-five pounds is a lot for us!"

No wonder women feel intimidated in the gym. The truth is, men are still not used to seeing women in "bro territory." They are as confused about us being there as we are about what to do with the equipment! But you and I have every right to enjoy lifting weights and be in the weight room just like any guy.

In hindsight, rather than meet annoyance with anger, I should have simply explained that I was in the middle of my sets and would be finished momentarily. It probably would have diffused his attitude.

Understanding how to use the equipment will make you feel more confident in the weight room. Then, it's just a matter of getting a few workouts under your belt to start feeling more comfortable there among the men. Now I spend most of my time in bro territory at the gym, and because of this, I have a ton of male friends there. Because they see that I am comfortable and happy to play nice with them, they treat me just like any other friend. A big part of getting comfortable amidst the sea of men is, simply, you getting comfortable.

Why are the rest phases so precise? Can't I just rest as long as I need to?

Rest phases do two things for you.

1. They give your muscles and overall system time to strategically recover so you can put the right amount of effort into your next set. Depending on the 90-day training program that you follow, I want you to enter each new set about 50 to 80 percent recovered. This way, you enter the set feeling strong. For example, I like Easy Gainers to enter a set only about 50 percent recovered, whereas I like Hard Gainers to enter a set around 80 percent recovered.

2. Rest phases keep you from getting too much recovery in between sets and exercises. If your rest phases are too long, your muscles will recover fully. This detracts from progressive resistance (increased intensity over time) and can actually reduce a muscle's ability to generate force. Too much rest also disrupts the cumulative fatigue that occurs over the course of the entire workout while adequate rest ensures you get the right results from your selected training program. Bottom line: Fatigue is essential to developing strength and muscle mass, so resting as long as you feel you need to can actually backfire.

What should I do if I start losing motivation?

Don't freak. It happens. Give yourself some slack. Sometimes lack of motivation is a subtle form of fatigue or overtraining. Do this:

1. Take 1 or 2 days off from exercise. If you once felt an enthusiasm about your workouts and now you're feeling more "blah," you might need a few days to regenerate your physical inspiration. Allow yourself some rest and see how you feel in a few days. Often, that's all it takes to get back in the swing.

2. Mix up your routine. If you normally exercise in the morning, try moving your workouts to the evening for a week or two. If you've been following one of the programs with strength and cardio workouts only, try adding in one new workout next week. Try yoga, Spinning, outdoor hiking, or a dance class. It's amazing what a new experience can do for your motivation. Human beings like variety—it's possible that your lackluster motivation is simply boredom.

3. Sit down with a journal and finish these four sentences.
    a. I started this fitness program because . . .
    b. I am feeling unmotivated today because . . .
    c. I know that if I take action and complete my scheduled workouts this week I will feel . . .
    d. I want to achieve my fitness goals because it will make me feel . . .
4. As you review what you wrote, remember these things.
    a. All progress in life requires new action. In order to be different, it is essential that you behave differently.
    b. Making your fitness program a priority demonstrates that you are making yourself a priority. Taking care of your commitments at work, at home, and with friends is important. You will be a better partner, friend, and parent if you prioritize some time for yourself.
    c. In order to achieve your goals, you absolutely must take action. Reconnect with all of the reasons that you started this journey—they are important.

If I get off track for a few weeks, do I have to start over? Where do I pick up and continue?

The ocean tides cycle in and out. Seasons change. Even your body has natural circadian rhythms that change during the day. It is absolutely normal and human to get off track in your fitness endeavors. The most important thing is to avoid getting frustrated. Life throws curveballs, and the best solution is to become good at getting back on track. If your 90-day program gets interrupted, it is super easy to jump back in. Here are some general guidelines for knowing where to pick up.

If you have been off track for 2 weeks or less: Simply pick up where you left off in your 90-day training plan. It will take 1 week of workouts for your body to get back on track physically. During this 1st week, you might want to lower your weight loads and increase your rest phases by 30 seconds. Then, repeat this same week of programming for your 2nd week back at the gym, but at the weight loads and rest phases that you were performing before your hiatus. After this 2nd week of workouts, you'll be back on track.

If you have been off track for more than 2 weeks: Return to the beginning of the month where you left off. For example, if your last workout was in the 3rd week of programming of the 2nd month of workouts, you'll return to the gym and follow the programming for the 1st week of Month 3. Additionally, you'll want to begin with lower weight loads than where you left off. You may also need to increase your rest phases by 30 seconds, depending on your level of de-training.

A business trip will take me away from home for 14 days. If I can't get to a gym, are there exercises I can do in my hotel that'll keep me in shape?

Here is a maintenance workout that you can do on the road: Complete the following exercises in order using just your body weight. Perform as many reps as you can in 1 minute for each exercise and then go immediately into the next exercise. Rest for 1 minute after you have completed all five exercises, before you begin the next round or circuit. Aim to complete 3 to 6 circuits depending on your time and fitness level. (These five exercises are explained in Chapter 7.)

Goblet Squat
Walking Lunge
All Fours Crunch
Bench Stepup
Bicycle

A Walk-Through for Your First Workout

Ladies, start your engines! Let's go step-by-step through a sample workout so that you'll look like an ace while you're still getting familiar with the gym. Prior to arriving at the gym, print out your 90-day training program of choice or have it on your smartphone so you have an outline of the workout ready to guide you.

Bring the book with you as a visual guide to help you perform the exercises correctly. Also, you ate something, right? And hydrated your body with water? Good. Strap on your sports watch and apply your game face.

For this example, let's use the Hard Gainer training program Workout A for legs, back, and abs—one of my favorites.

The Warmup

Once you leave the locker room, head for a piece of cardio equipment. It doesn't matter which one—stationary bike, treadmill, rowing machine, elliptical. Just use what's available. Hop on and start out slowly, gradually easing into higher levels of intensity. Do this for 6 to 10 minutes, so that by the end you are feeling a bit sweaty and nicely energized, not fatigued.

The Workout

Find your way to the leg curl machine. Pause for a moment to check and see if anyone else appears to be using it. If not, all systems go!

Make adjustments to the machine based on your height and estimated workload. If you are brand new to strength training, you'll need to take a stab at your starting weight load. In the beginning, it's a bit of a guessing game, and that's okay! Over time you will become more familiar with your starting workloads for all equipment. A good rule of thumb is to start conservative and go light. Technique is so important and a lighter weight load will allow you to assess the three steps to strength from Chapter 6. Then, you'll have a better sense of where your current abilities are.

Here, again, are some suggested starting weight loads.

Leg Curl—30 to 40 pounds
Leg Press—50 to 70 pounds
Reverse Grip Pulldown—30 to 50 pounds
Goblet Squat—20 to 30 pounds
Bent-Over Barbell Row—30 to 40 pounds
Walking Lunge—0 (body weight only) to 10 pounds

Leg Extension—20 to 50 pounds

Seated Upright Chest Fly—20 to 40 pounds

Barbell Overhead Press—20 to 30 pounds

Dumbbell Bent Arm Side Raise—5 to 8 pounds

Dumbbell Hammer Curl—5 to 10 pounds

Dumbbell French Press—5 to 8 pounds

Calf Raise—20 to 30 pounds

Foolproof Weight

If your last 2 reps were perfect, it's time to bump up the weight load. Can you say "rock star"? The general rule of thumb is:

A 10-pound increase for lower-body exercises

A 5-pound increase for upper-body exercises

When you're ready to begin a set, be sure to review the exercise instruction in the book. Pay attention to the tips for good form. Are your feet positioned properly? Are your abs drawn inward but still allowing a natural arch in your lower back? Are your shoulders back and down?

As you begin the set, feel out the first 5 or 6 repetitions. You'll be able to tell if the weight is way too heavy, way too light, or maybe somewhere in between. This "somewhere in between" is the sweet spot. If those first reps feel way too heavy, simply stop the set, change the weight, rest for 30 seconds, and start again. It's always fine to have one or two sets that serve as a warmup before you find the right weight load for that exercise. Let Step 3 (last 2 reps) really guide you here.

Perform the first set for 12 reps using the Three-Step System to Strength, focusing on an enthusiastic Hard phase, a pause at the point of maximal effort, and a slow Easy phase. Make sure you're breathing! As soon as you finish your 12 reps, start your stopwatch for your 60-second rest. During your rest period take a sip of water and quickly assess the quality of the last 2 reps of your set. Were they easy with perfect form? If so, you want to increase the weight load on this machine by 5 to 10 pounds for your second set. If the last 2 reps of your set were a wee bit sloppy, keep the current weight and see what happens on your second set. If you struggled to complete the entire first set of 12 reps and were unable to maintain excellent technique, you can feel confident in lowering the weight. Remember, technique trumps all! If your technique wasn't great, let your ego take a walk and go ahead and lower your weight load.

Okay, 60 seconds is up! Let's get into your second set. Perform this set for 12 reps using the Three-Step System to Strength. Once you complete your reps, start your stopwatch. Quickly assess your performance and make a note regarding the weight loads that worked for this exercise today as you rest. Then, it's time to get going on to the next movement: Leg Press.

One quick thing to note, though: Be mindful of your rest-phase time. Even though you are moving on to a new exercise, you still want to try and respect the designated rest phase; don't allow for it to go too long. It might take you a bit longer to move on to the machine and get it ready for your set, so take that into consideration. Just try to keep moving and stay within the designated rest time as much as possible.

Now you're ready for the Leg Press. Review the exercise description and performance pointers. Do your feet look symmetrically placed on the footplate? Is your lower back in position? Perform 15 reps using the Three-Step System to Strength, and start your stopwatch when you are finished.

During your 60 seconds of rest, assess the weight load and your performance. How were the last 2 reps of that set? Need to make changes to your workload? If so, hop to it so that you can be ready in 60 seconds. If you do need to make weight adjustments, remember that 10 pounds is a good weight change for leg exercises. If your set was great, you can hang out and ponder life and get ready for the second Leg Press set.

Next, you've got 60 seconds to make your way to the lat pulldown machine and get set up. You rush on over, put down your towel, and select your starting weight load. And then—a cute but snarling dude comes over and says, "I was using that machine." See, it happens sometimes! He wandered off for a drink of water and you snagged the machine! You've got two options.

1. Tell him you'll be quick because you only have two sets.
2. Smile sweetly, apologize, and ask if you can work in with him.

Most likely he'll be happy to share the machine with you. And everyone will live happily ever after. I think you're getting the drift here. Continue through your workout in the same exact manner as the example above.

Easy Gainers, Listen Up!

If you are going to be following the Easy Gainer program, you'll be using super-sets and won't have dedicated rest phases in between exercises. In this case, the sets are just a bit different. For example, for Workout A you'll begin with one Leg Press set then immediately go to your first Reverse Grip Pulldown set. After that, you'll start your stopwatch for your first 30-second rest phase as you make your way back to the leg press machine. You'll then repeat that same superset of Leg Press and Reverse Grip Pulldown for your second set. After these two super-sets, you'll move on to the Walking Lunge and Bent-Over Barbell Row superset during your 30-second rest phase.

Wow! Time flies when you're having fun. That's all you need to know in order to have a stupendous first workout. You are now officially an expert. You go, girl!

Don't Be Shy: Use the Mirrors

The mirrors in the gym are there for a reason, and it's not so you can touch up your hair or admire your derriere. Use them to check your form and become a technician of body awareness. Another term for body awareness is *proprioception*. It's your ability to know where your body is in space without looking. A strong sense of body awareness leads to symmetry in how you use the right and left sides of your body during an exercise, and watching yourself in the mirrors is the best way to do that. For example, during the Dumbbell Bent Arm Side Raise exercise, check the mirror to make sure that both arms are rising equally high, that both elbows hold the same angle, and that the dumbbells end in an equal position. If you don't see that symmetry reflected in the mirror, you risk developing muscle imbalances that can lead to injury. Reflect on that for a bit and use those mirrors!

Chapter 14
Booster Rockets for Faster Results

Once you have the workouts down, there's lots more you can do to achieve the strong, healthy, energetic body you're after. An exceptional fitness level requires an exceptional lifestyle. What you do in between workouts influences your rate of progress, ease of recovery, and general well-being. This chapter will outline a few ways to complement your training program and achieve even better results.

Add Cardio into the Mix

Your cardiovascular system is responsible for supplying your body with oxygen to fuel movement. Cardiovascular fitness reflects how well your heart and lungs do their job and how well your muscles use the oxygen. The concept of cardiovascular exercise (cardio) has gotten very diluted and misused. There are very specific reasons for doing cardio. The problem is that most people lump all cardio together and think that hopping on the treadmill will meet their cardio needs. Just like with other areas of fitness, it's important to be strategic in how and why you do cardio.

The 90-day training programs in this book do not stipulate cardio workouts. That's because this is a book about strength training and I didn't want to take the emphasis away from what I feel deserves your full attention. However, without a doubt, cardio is important for good health and getting lean. Here are some great cardio activities to add into your strength-training program.

> Brisk walking

> Running

> Cycling

> Swimming

> Using cardio machines (elliptical or stair climber)

> Spinning

> Rowing

> Aerobic dancing

The effectiveness of cardio workouts is completely dependent on the intensity, which is a reflection of your heart rate. To keep things simple, I suggest steady-state cardio. This means that you will engage in your activity of choice at a consistent intensity level for the length of the workout. Trainers call this beta-oxidation cardio; it specifically utilizes stored body fat as the primary source of fuel for your muscles during the session. This kind of cardio is in contrast to interval training, where you intentionally change the levels during your workout to make your heart rate go up and down. While there is certainly a time and place for interval training, I tend to recommend steady-state cardio most of the time because it is straightforward, pleasurable, and reduces carbohydrate cravings. Women process carbohydrates differently than men and tend to respond best to steady-state, beta-oxidation cardio. Interval-training sessions can make women ravenous and cause them to consume more calories than the workout burns off, thus canceling out the effort.

In order to fine-tune your cardio workouts and keep that from happening, you can estimate your heart rate using the RPE Scale, which stands for "rating of

RPE Scale

0	Nothing at all	5	Strong
0.5	Very, very weak	6	Strong
1	Very weak	7	Very strong
2	Weak	8	Very strong
3	Moderate	9	Very strong
4	Somewhat strong	10	Very, very strong; maximal

perceived exertion." This scale will help to ensure that your heart rate is in line with your cardio goals. Above you will see my intensity recommendation for each kind of cardio based on your goal. To use this scale, make a quick assessment of how hard you are working during your cardio session. You will rate your perceived exertion on a scale from 1 to 10, where 1 reflects what you would feel when you are really relaxed, like resting on the couch, and 10 reflects what you would feel if you engaged in an incredibly strenuous activity, like running as fast as possible. At any given moment during your cardio workout, summarize your overall effort level and rate it on the scale. Recognizing your level of exertion will help you to maintain the proper pace for your goal.

Adding a cardio workout to your strength-training program can improve your muscles' adaptation to strength training, decrease body fat, boost cardiovascular health, facilitate recovery, and improve general physical conditioning. Here are five specific benefits of cardio and how to build each into your 90-day program.

1. **Help muscles adapt and use carbs more efficiently.** Aim for three or four 25-minute sessions per week at an RPE level of 5.

2. **Accelerate fat loss.** Aim for four to six 35-minute sessions per week at an RPE of 4.

3. **Strengthen the heart.** The heart is a muscle that needs progressive resistance just like other muscles, so aim for four 30-minute cardio sessions per week at an RPE of 7 to 8.

4. **Speed recovery from tough strength-training sessions.** Light cardio increases bloodflow to your muscles to flush in nutrients and flush out damage from workouts. Cardio for recovery can be done after your strength workouts, or on separate days. Aim for three 20-minute sessions per week at a low intensity, such as an RPE of 3.

5. **Improve general fitness and conditioning.** This is helpful if you are training for an event or other sport, since it improves endurance and overall resilience. Aim for three to five 30-minute sessions per week at an RPE between 4 and 5.

You should strategically schedule your cardio workouts based on your strength-training goals. If you are determined to increase lean muscle mass, schedule your cardio workouts after your strength-training sessions, or hold them for a separate day. You don't want to perform a full cardio workout prior to your strength workouts because you want to reserve your energy for the strength session. This applies especially if you are following the Hard Gainer and Radical Transformation programs.

However, if you know that you gain muscle easily and want to focus on building strength, rather than increasing lean muscle mass, schedule your cardio workouts immediately prior to your strength sessions. This pre-fatigues your system so that you will have less energy to put into your strength workout and makes it even harder to increase lean muscle mass. This applies if you are following the Easy Gainer program.

And if you are brand new to strength training, or are returning to the gym after an extended hiatus, reserve any cardio sessions for days when you are not strength training. This applies if you are following the Newbie or Hard Gainer program.

Don't Be Afraid to Eat

Some women feel they should starve themselves to lose weight. That's just flawed thinking. When you deprive yourself of nutrition, your body starts to attack muscle to fuel its necessary functions. You will burn off excess body fat and build lean, strong muscle by eating four to six times a day and making sure to include a combination of protein, fat, and carbohydrates at every meal or snack. Here are an outline for each meal and some suggestions.

Breakfast: Protein is extra important at breakfast. Aim for 15 to 25 grams of protein from sources like eggs, egg whites, protein powders, or lean meats. Combine this with slow-digesting carbs like whole grains, berries, or beans. Be sure to add some healthy fats like avocado, olive oil, or nut butter.

Lunch: A salad full of colorful vegetables and topped with some protein—like chicken, turkey, or tuna (or vegetarian sources of protein like tofu or beans)—makes a great meal. You're in luck: Choose low-fat salad dressing instead of fat-free. You need some fat in all of your meals for satiety and hormone production. Aim for 18 to 20 grams of protein, lots of filling vegetables, and just a dash of salad dressing.

Snacks: Keeping your blood sugar stable means fewer cravings, energy slumps, and mood swings. Avoid going longer than 4 hours without a meal or snack. Try a few slices of deli turkey, a hard-cooked egg, or low-fat Greek yogurt for protein. Pair this with whole grain crackers, hummus, or berries. In a pinch, I sometimes grab a healthy protein bar. These are all great snacks to eat before your workout as well.

Dinner: Here, too, it's important to combine good sources of protein with carbs and fat. Great options are broiled salmon with broccoli and brown rice; grilled chicken with olive oil and grilled asparagus; or a salad made with tomatoes, cucumbers, bell peppers, cheese chunks, and pieces of rotisserie chicken. Planning dinner shouldn't be difficult. My mantra is: "Protein, green vegetables, and some healthy fat." If I'm really hungry, I'll add in a baked sweet potato.

It's worth repeating how important it is to properly fuel up after a workout. While you might think you are doing yourself a favor by denying your body calories in order to lose weight, realize that your tank is pretty much empty after a good workout. And there is a very special window of opportunity after exercise when your body is primed to use calories and nutrients for recovery.

This is an often-overlooked consideration that seriously affects your results. What you eat—or don't eat—after your workout determines how quickly and effectively you recover. There is a very direct correlation between your post-workout refueling and the quality of your next workout.

For many years I was operating under the notion that the goal of a workout was to burn calories in order to lose weight. Therefore, I would often go into my workouts empty and not eat afterward until I was hungry. It made sense to me: Why eat when the whole goal is to burn off calories? And during those years, I saw very little improvement in my fitness, was sore all the time, and never felt energized. How you eat after your workout influences:

> Muscular adaptation

> Muscle soreness

> The quality of subsequent workouts

> Appetite and food cravings

> Mood

In the simplest terms, your muscles need protein and carbohydrates in order to repair the "damage" from your workout. If you don't feed your body properly, your muscles will be unable to repair themselves, which means chronic muscle soreness. Your muscles will be in a state of continual repair, so you won't be powered and energized for your workouts. In order to catch up and repair, your muscles will demand carbohydrates. You'll feel chronically fatigued and maybe even overcompensate on carbs when the cravings kick in, resulting in weight gain.

Your first line of defense is to be strategic in how and what you eat after your training sessions. Most research shows that the window of opportunity is wide open for 60 minutes after a workout. During this time, your body will gladly gobble up what you give it and shuttle it to your muscles for repair. In some circles, it is a practice to use this window for a "cheat meal." Your body will use the food to literally refuel your muscles and liver back to their full levels. In theory, you're able to eat extra calories and have some fun with your food choices during this window with few negative repercussions. (Hello sugar! Howdy fat!)

I think it's a much smarter strategy to choose healthy foods that can be absorbed quickly, like easily digested proteins and carbohydrates. And the sooner you eat after your workout, the better. The window may be open for 60 minutes, but it's wider immediately after your workout. I suggest eating right away, as you walk out of the gym, if possible.

The name of the game after a tough workout is to choose fast-digesting carbs paired with easily digestible protein. This is the time when you want to avoid fat as much as possible. Here are some good protein and carb options for after your workout.

Proteins

Fat-free milk

Plain Greek yogurt

Protein powders

Egg whites

Carbs

Tropical fruit

Honey

White potatoes

Fruit juice

White bread

Sugar

Take Rest Days Seriously

Your rest days are just as important as, if not more important than, your strength-training days because that's when the muscle repair happens. If you are just getting back into exercise, take 2 to 3 days off from exercise altogether each week. If you have a longer history of consistent exercise, you should be able to benefit from 5 to 6 days of activity, allowing for 1 day of complete rest each week. Even professional athletes take at least 1 day off from exercise every week. Be sure to schedule your day off and do nothing very physical. Just veg.

In each of the four 90-day programs, I've built in 3 consecutive rest days before beginning the next 27-day period. These are designed to allow your body a deeper level of recovery. Don't skip them. There is a cumulative effect of fatigue that can slowly and quietly creep up on you. One day you think you're doing just fine, and then bam, you get a cold, notice weird aches and pains, or find that you are chronically sore from workouts. At some point, the body will demand rest if you don't allow for some concentrated recovery time after several weeks of training.

During these 3 days each month, you have a choice. You can take these days off completely from exercise, or you can engage in very light recovery activities. You will see best results from this program if you get the most from these days of recovery. Therefore, take an assessment of your fatigue at the end of each 27-day cycle. If you are feeling totally pooped from the workouts, enjoy your 3 days of laziness. If you are feeling energized after your 27 days, consider active recovery activities for your days off, such as:

> Leisurely walking
> Gardening
> Light stretching
> Social dancing
> Restorative yoga

Remember: Your days of rest are just as important as your days of exercise.

Deal with DOMS

DOMS stands for delayed onset muscle soreness, and it occurs from microtears in the muscle fibers as a result of new or strenuous exercise. Low-level damage like this is essential to change your muscles in order to help you get lean. In some ways, muscle soreness is a positive thing because it indicates that you taxed your muscles beyond their current ability, and this initiates change and growth. Most people experience soreness 24 to 48 hours after a strength-training session. I pretty much always feel it within 24 hours after my workout, but I have clients who feel it 48 hours after. I also have some clients who never get sore, even after extremely hard workouts. Just like everything else, muscle soreness is a personalized experience. It's important to recognize that muscle soreness is not a prerequisite for change. While its presence is a clear sign that you taxed your muscles, it is possible to make great progress with little to no soreness. The most important factor in changing your muscles is taxing them beyond their current ability and then allowing them to recover. This can occur with or without muscle soreness.

Even highly trained athletes experience soreness after they have engaged in a new activity. And you will most likely experience muscle soreness simply because of your new workouts. There are two kinds of soreness to be aware of. There is the kind where you wake up in the morning and feel like your muscles have been used and are fatigued. I love this feeling! Makes me feel accomplished! Then there is the other kind of soreness, where standing up and sitting down are misery. Most likely this occurs from pushing yourself too hard in your workout. I see this happen with new clients. Either they are the personality type who like to push themselves very hard, or they are overcaffeinating before workouts. Caffeine is a great tool for fitness, but it does serve as an analgesic (pain reducer). This means that you might push harder than your body is technically prepared for. I see great results when I have clients cut back on caffeine. This allows them to work at an effort level that accurately reflects their fitness abilities.

Intense soreness can also occur after you performed a movement that had extended time under tension during the Easy phase. The Walking Lunge exercise is a perfect example. There is a longer Easy phase as you lower toward the floor that causes more damage to the muscle. Consider this a warning: If you are new to this exercise, be sure to start with just your body weight and stick with the number of sets and reps noted in your program.

Here are some ways that you can manage muscle soreness.

Assess your level of fatigue. You should feel tired and "worked" but not completely wrecked from your workout. If you feel completely wrecked, ease up during the next workout and see if that improves things.

Do some light cardio after your workout. Try 10 minutes of brisk walking or stationary cycling or do exactly what you did for your preworkout warmup. This helps to bring bloodflow to your muscles and can reduce soreness. Another good idea: foam-rolling.

Eat protein after a workout. Some research suggests that eating fast-digesting protein after workouts can help to minimize soreness. I've had great success with my clients who've tried this. I see a very real correlation with soreness and improper refueling. I pretty much never miss a postworkout "meal" that emphasizes protein.

Take a few extra days off. Overtraining can result from poor recovery, rather than from intense workouts. If you find that you are chronically sore even after troubleshooting with the tips above, you may need more time off in between workouts. In this case, take 2 to 3 days off from exercise altogether and reassess 2 weeks later.

Ice, ice, baby! Ice reigns supreme when it comes to muscle soreness. At the onset of muscle soreness, ice the area for 8 to 10 minutes, two to three times per day, until soreness subsides. The best way is to use real ice, placed in a waterproof bag directly on the skin. You don't have to worry about frostbite when using real ice, but it's wise to avoid using reusable ice packs for this reason. If the soreness is substantial—like, can't-sit-down substantial—anti-inflammatories like ibuprofen are great when used immediately before bed.

Chapter 15
Lift to Get Lean Grocery List

Fuel your workouts with these healthy staples

Take a time-out from the weight room for a minute. Outside the gym are two more essential places you'll want to get to know better on your journey to get lean: the grocery store and your kitchen. Just as a sports car needs high-octane fuel, your muscles require premium ingredients to perform at their peak. After all, there's a reason they're called muscle cars! So speed right by the fast food, and reroute your trip to your favorite grocery store, where you'll stock up on the best fresh foods available to make meals at home. You don't want to miss the benefits of the nutritional powerhouse foods we'll review in this chapter.

But before we get to the grocery list, let me tackle a question I'm always asked by friends and clients: "How should I eat?" What does a perfect day of eating look like?

That's really tough to answer because so much depends on your personal preferences and goals, but there are some general guidelines that anyone can use to set out on the right path for fueling the body properly to maximize the workouts in this book.

A Perfect Day of Eating

You don't have to be rigid about timing your meals; you can be flexible—just try to avoid going longer than 4 hours without eating a meal or snack. If you want a more specific answer, try this plan designed to provide a steady stream of energy to your muscles and keep your blood sugar levels stable so you don't become ravenous during the day, which can lead to craving-fueled binges. And remember this one very important guideline: Incorporate some protein, healthy carbohydrates, and fats into every meal or snack.

Breakfast: The morning meal is important because you are "breaking the fast." You've been fasting for the past 8 to 12 hours, mostly while asleep. Your metabolism—your body's furnace—has throttled down, and now your brain and muscles crave a healthy dose of high-quality protein and carbohydrates. Numerous studies back up what mothers have been saying for decades: "Eat your breakfast!" One famed study at Virginia Commonwealth University found that dieters who regularly ate a protein-rich, full breakfast lost significantly more weight (and kept it off longer) than another group who ate a low-calorie morning meal with a quarter of the protein.

The ideal breakfast is high in protein—eggs are a great choice—to keep you satiated and packed with slow-burning, fiber-rich vegetables and whole grains (to prevent blood sugar swings). A two-egg omelet with chopped broccoli, spinach, or yellow bell peppers paired with whole grain bread or oatmeal is an ideal way to start the day because it gives you each of those important macronutrients: protein, healthy carbs, and fats.

Midmorning Snack: Kill 10:30 a.m. cravings with a high-quality protein, such as that found in Greek yogurt. The more protein you eat early on, the longer you'll feel full throughout the day. I suggest adding some fresh berries to the yogurt, for sweetness and fiber—maybe a tablespoon of ground flaxseeds, too.

Lunch: This is a great opportunity to fill up on vegetables. Many of us don't want to eat heavy at lunch because it weighs us down and makes us tired in the afternoon. That's why a big salad is a good choice. Shoot for a salad made with at least three vegetables besides the base greens and include some quality proteins (fish, poultry, beef, or tofu) and healthy fats from an olive-oil-based dressing. Since the veggies are mainly water, fiber, and vitamins, they will keep you hydrated and your belly full of healthy calories. If you are having a sandwich for lunch, start out with a side salad. Research shows that kicking off your lunch with a salad helps slow digestion so that you don't overeat.

Afternoon Snack: To avoid the pangs that send some of us hunting for the nearest vending machine, bring healthy snacks to work with you. A handful of almonds and a handful of fresh red grapes are all it takes to ward off cravings and keep your mind focused on your work. Other good choices: $\frac{1}{2}$ cup of low-fat cottage cheese, a banana with a tablespoon of almond butter or natural peanut butter, a piece of string cheese, or a slice of turkey breast lunchmeat rolled up with a slice of Swiss cheese. And if you work out after work and before dinner, add a protein shake with some carbohydrates in it to fuel your exercise.

Dinner: This meal can be dangerous to your belly if you aren't careful. Eating too much at dinner has the tendency to ignite your appetite and cause you to overeat late at night. That's why I recommend going light for the evening meal— something like stir-fried shrimp with vegetables and brown rice, and a dessert of fresh fruit salad. Eating low-calorie, high-fiber vegetables will decrease your overall food intake by 10 percent or more. And the shrimp will provide lean protein and heart-healthy omega-3s. The fruit salad is a sweet way to end the meal and it delivers a bowlful of anti-inflammatory vitamins.

Evening Snack: You can do without this snack. It's certainly not mandatory, but if you have the munchies or need a little help falling asleep, try a medium banana and 6 ounces of kefir. Bananas have a satisfying creamy texture and contain melatonin, a natural sleep-regulating hormone, in addition to potassium and calcium, which may help lower blood pressure. The kefir contains tryptophan, an amino acid that has a relaxing effect on the nervous system.

Keeping their fuel tank filled throughout the day often helps people manage their blood sugar better to avoid the peaks and valleys that trigger overeating. For that reason, you may find the above guidelines helpful. *What* to eat is another part of the equation. I gave you a few suggestions. Your options for healthy fare are almost limitless. Next, I'm going to give you a grocery list of my

My Go-To Postworkout Snacks

Low-fat dairy is my favorite bet after a workout because it delivers protein to your muscles very quickly. If I can't grab a protein shake, I'll choose other low-fat dairy products. Yogurt's protein-to-carb ratio helps stabilize blood sugar and support muscle breakdown and recovery. My favorite is Fage Strawberry Goji, which contains 120 calories, no fat, 17 grams of carbs, and 13 grams of protein. Chocolate milk delivers protein to your muscles quickly, plus a little bit of sugar to restore liver and muscle glycogen. For low-fat chocolate milk, I like Horizon Organic Chocolate Lowfat Milk with DHA Omega-3. Thanks to its ideal balance of protein and carbs, chocolate moo juice has been shown to help assist recovery after a workout. And this carton is fortified with omega-3s to make sure your brain doesn't feel left out. One cup delivers 160 calories, 2.4 grams of fat, 26 grams of carbs, and 9 grams of protein. It's an excellent substitute for a sports drink.

go-to superfoods (plus some quick options if you're in a pinch) to build your own meal plan. You'll notice that almost all are fresh whole foods rather than processed and packaged items. Stick with these and follow my guidelines on portion and calorie control and you'll keep your metabolism firing on all cylinders to achieve your hottest bod yet.

Here, in alphabetical order, are some of the most healthful foods to be had—they fight fat, stoke your metabolism, deliver optimum energy, boost your immune system, and ward off the ravages of aging and disease. And, oh yeah, very importantly: They taste great!

Agave Nectar

There's a time and a place for tequila, though it's probably best to avoid downing that use of the agave plant every day. But raw blue agave nectar is a great sugar (or honey) substitute to try in your tea, yogurt, or protein shake. Agave nectar tastes

If you find that you are craving snacks in the evening, take a hard look at what you're eating in the morning for breakfast. In a study at the University of Missouri, women who started their day with a protein-rich meal like eggs consumed 135 fewer snack calories after dinner. The researchers say a protein-heavy first meal prevents the secretion of the hunger hormone ghrelin and stimulates the release of the satiety hormone peptide YY, leading to less hunger in the evening.

sweeter than honey or sugar, so use it sparingly! One tablespoon contains less sugar and fewer calories and carbohydrates than honey—not to mention that it has a lower glycemic index, giving you more stable energy without the nasty spikes.

Almonds

I like to keep a handful of almonds with me in case of a hunger emergency. Packed with protein, fiber, calcium, and iron, they're easy to grab on the go to ward off my midmorning stomach growls. Plus, researchers from Pennsylvania State University reported that people who ate 1.5 ounces of almonds a day for 6 weeks were able to reduce their belly fat and waist circumference and lower their LDL (bad) cholesterol.

Apples

Don't want to gain a bushel? Then eat more apples. Scientists at the University of Iowa found that a compound known as ursolic acid that is found in apples increased metabolism-revving muscle mass and boosted levels of brown fat (which burns other fat) in lab mice. The findings could eventually lead to a supplement potent enough to have the same effect in humans. In the meantime, chomp away—apples can also suppress your appetite and help whittle your tummy. And not only do they deliver a satisfying crunch and filling fiber, but this A-list fruit has also been linked with improving overall sexual function for women and warding off obesity-related disorders. Research published in the *Archives of Gynecology and Obstetrics* reported that the health-hiking polyphenols in apples' skin may improve bloodflow below the belt, aiding in more satisfying sex.

Arugula

Nothing personal against salads built on the usual leafy bed of iceberg lettuce heads, but arugula contains about twice as much bone-building calcium and magnesium. Plus its peppery taste packs just the right kick of flavor. Other ways to extend your leafy green repertoire? Eat more romaine and red leaf lettuce, spinach, watercress, endive, Swiss chard, and radicchio. For an easy path to these more uncharted greens, pick up a package of spring mix, which may contain all of the above.

Asparagus

Your tongue may be one of the strongest muscles in your body, but another organ is more in control of your life: your brain. So why not boost your brain function with folate-rich asparagus? In addition, it is one of the richest sources of rutin, a compound that strengthens capillary walls (blood vessels), and a 5.3-ounce serving harbors 3 grams of dietary fiber. Plus, it's a 5-minute add-on to any meal. Swipe the spears with a dash of olive oil, grill them for 5 or 6 minutes (turning to avoid any charring), and top with cracked black pepper and sea salt.

Avocado

This tasty and versatile craving-killer is A-list material for warding off mid-morning or midafternoon hunger pangs. According to research published in *Nutrition Journal*, adding half an avocado to your lunch can decrease your desire to munch between meals by 40 percent. Add sliced or chopped avocados to any meal: Serve them alongside eggs, sprinkle them on a salad or atop chicken, or blend them into a smoothie.

Bananas

Bananas contain a type of dietary fiber known as resistant starch that your body can't absorb, so they fill you up without filling you out. Resistant starch is also

Chip Shots

Outsmart cravings with these wise swaps

Often when you crave a food it's the texture that you are hankering for—crunchy, creamy, greasy, or fluid. When a certain texture calls your name more than your waistband would like, use these smart swaps to help you satisfy the craving without adding inches.

When you crave: crunchy foods (chips, caramel popcorn, biscotti)

Swap in this: whole grain crackers with hummus, or caramel rice cakes with a thin spread of nut butter, or ¼ cup freshly toasted pecans drizzled with agave and a tiny sprinkle of salt (my fave!)

When you crave: creamy foods (peanut butter, risotto, mac 'n' cheese)

Swap in this: sugar-free gelatin, hummus, whey protein pudding, or, for dinner, a bowl of velvety tomato or squash soup

When you crave: greasy foods (fries, pizza, burgers)

Swap in this: baked sweet potato fries, thin-crust pizza with veggies, or a 90 percent lean beef burger—your mouth won't know the difference

When you crave: fluids (juice, soda, slushies)

Swap in this: flavored sparkling water or lightly sweetened iced tea. (Studies suggest that limiting caloric beverages leads to weight loss.) Or try a smoothie. Research shows that the thicker and more whipped the drink, the more satisfying it will be, saving you calories at your next meal. To achieve maximum thickness, toss in a frozen banana and blend.

linked with an increase in postmeal fat-burning. One of the by-products of the unabsorbed carbohydrates in your system is butyrate, a fatty acid that may inhibit the body's ability to burn carbs, forcing your metabolism to focus on incinerating fat instead. What's more, research from The Smell and Taste Treatment and Research Foundation in Chicago reported the smell of bananas helps reduce appetite, so you may not want to eat as much anyway.

Beans and Legumes

Slow-digesting carbohydrates win the race to deliver dietary fiber and protein to your daily menu. Here's which ones are worthy of top billing.

Black beans: They're rich in an antioxidant called anthocyanin, which fights heart disease and cancer.

Chickpeas: (garbanzo beans): In one study, a chickpea-fortified diet slashed bad cholesterol levels by 5 percent. Toss them into salads or mash them up and blend them with garlic for homemade hummus.

Navy beans: These guys pack enough potassium to regulate blood pressure and keep your heart rate contractions normal.

Pinto beans: Pintos are filled with fiber to help stabilize blood sugar and lower your risk of type 2 diabetes.

Beef

It's a prime source of protein, but it's also rich in two key muscle-building nutrients: iron and zinc. As a natural source of creatine, beef also boosts your energy supply for time you spend at the gym. Save marble for your countertops and choose a leaner cut of beef like rounds or loins from the meat aisle.

Beets

These crimson crusaders are a serious source of folate and betaine—two nutrients that work in tandem to lower your blood levels of homocysteine, an inflammatory compound that can damage your arteries and increase your risk of heart disease. Opt for raw, fresh beets instead of their canned cousins. Boil, peel, and chop them to use as a salad topper or brighten up a stew.

Bell Peppers

Besides adding a pop of color (and crunch) to your plate, green, red, yellow, and orange bell peppers are all great sources of vitamin C, vitamin B_6, and folate. But there's more than meets the eye—the phytochemicals that give peppers their bright shades also protect you from heart disease, cancer, stroke, and cataracts.

Berries

Blueberries: Aim for $\frac{1}{2}$ cup of these babies a day. If you're buying in bulk, try tossing a handful in the freezer as a stand-in for frozen treats—blueberries are just as nutritious frozen as they are fresh and don't come with any of the guilt ice cream does. According to the USDA, one particular antioxidant found in these tiny berries—anthocyanin—can stimulate liver cells to break down fat and cholesterol better and fight off inflammation. The darker the berry, the better the bennies.

Cranberries: These tiny red berries bring more antioxidants to the table than all other common fruits except blueberries (thus their seeding here). Cranberries are also known as a natural probiotic, enhancing good bacteria levels in your gut and balancing your pH levels below the belt.

Strawberries, raspberries, and blackberries: This trio contains ellagic acid and a large number of polyphenols, which inhibit tumor growth. Raspberries and blackberries are loaded with fiber—8 grams in just 1 cup.

Bison

Beef gets all the glory, but a 3-ounce serving of the other red meat contains 5 more grams of protein, 32 fewer calories, and 3 fewer grams of fat. Trade your usual beef patties for bison, for a leaner protein that delivers just as much juicy flavor.

Black Tea

Think of black tea as the little black dress of beverages—universal, tasteful, and great for any occasion. Drink it hot in the a.m. to start your day with a dose of cholesterol-lowering catechins. Brew a bunch of tea bags and stow your iced tea in the fridge for a few days. Replace sugary sodas and diet drinks full of artificial sweeteners with unsweetened black tea, and you'll eliminate junk calories and harmful ingredients that weigh you down.

Broccoli

This vegetable provides one of the most powerful plant-based sources of nutrients for preventing the diseases of aging. Broccoli (and its sister cruciferous vegetables cauliflower, Brussels sprouts, and cabbage) contains abundant amounts of the antioxidant compound sulforaphane, which has been shown to prevent cancer and remove toxins from cells. Broccoli is also a good source of vitamin C, fiber, folate, vitamin D, vitamin B_6, folic acid, and the antioxidant quercetin, which has been associated with preventing age-related memory decline. It doesn't matter how you eat broccoli—steamed, sautéed, stir-fried, or raw—this powerhouse veggie delivers a boatload of benefits. And you don't always need fresh broccoli florets to enjoy those bennies. Stock up on frozen broccoli spears and florets—they are just as nutritious as fresh ones—to top your salads, toss into stir-fry dishes, and serve as a side with chicken or beef. Sprinkle grated Parmesan cheese on top or add a dab of butter; the fat will help your body better absorb the nutrients inside.

Brown Rice

It's simple: The milling and polishing that convert brown rice into white destroy the good-for-you vitamins this grain has to offer. But with brown rice, since only the outermost kernel is stripped away, you get the full benefits of fiber, thiamin, niacin, vitamin B$_6$, magnesium, and iron this mighty grain has to offer. Half a cup will only set you back 100 calories and is a great addition to any lean protein and vegetable to craft a well-rounded meal.

Brussels Sprouts

The arch-nemesis of your 8-year-old self is actually the hero of your new diet. One cup contains 4 grams of fiber and more than 100 percent of your daily allowance of vitamins C and K. Plus, cruciferous veggies like Brussels sprouts, broccoli, and kale contain compounds believed to flush cancer-causing toxins from your body. Still not sold? Try Maple-Glazed Brussels Sprouts (see recipe on page 243), or dip them in fondue for a calcium boost.

Cheese

Eliminating cheese is an easy way to clear out extra calories from a sandwich or a giant plate of nachos, but when you're in a pinch, a part-skim mozzarella cheese stick provides just the right amount of calcium, calories, and protein. Research published in the *British Journal of Nutrition* reported that people who ate a high-protein, moderate-calorie cheese snack ate less during their next meal. Avoid the fluorescent varieties and stick with part-skim mozzarella, mascarpone (a great substitute for butter), ricotta (a delicious dessert topping on fruit), and 1% milk fat cottage cheese (½ cup contains 14 grams of protein but fewer than 100 calories!).

Chicken

It's easy, lean, and pairs well with almost anything. A 4-ounce serving of chicken is the protein-powered champion, with about 36 grams of protein and just under 200 calories. Chicken is a complete protein, containing all of the essential amino acids your body requires on a daily basis, which is especially important in supporting your muscles as you strength train. The Institute of Medicine recommends women should aim for about 46 grams of protein per day—double that if they're exercising regularly, according to the International Society of Sports Nutrition.

Cinnamon

Fragrant, spicy cinnamon is rich in antioxidants that inhibit blood clotting and bacterial growth. But the most exciting thing about cinnamon is that studies show that it may help stabilize blood sugar, reducing the risk of type 2 diabetes. Sprinkle it on your oatmeal and more!

Cucumbers

Cucumber slices might look silly plastered on your eyes, but there's no joking about the hydrating, nutrient-rich properties of these vegetables. While applying them to the skin allows phytochemicals to tighten collagen for a firmer complexion, reducing the appearance of cellulite, there are also great benefits to eating them. Cucumber peel contains silica, an essential ingredient in wrinkle-preventing collagen. Stick with organic varieties to avoid the waxy coatings used to prolong shelf life.

Dark Chocolate

Research has shown that after a dark chocolate indulgence, women often feel two emotions: joy and guilt. Yikes. Here's all the justification you need to quit feeling guilty and enjoy a tasty bit of heaven every once in a while.

The antioxidants in cocoa, called polyphenols, can help increase bloodflow to your brain, improving your memory and alertness. Epicatechin, one of the compounds that gives cocoa its little bit of bitterness, can lower your blood pressure, easing your stress levels and cutting your stroke risk by 20 percent. Epicatechin also amplifies your cells' mitochondrial function, lending you surges of sustainable energy—and the darker the chocolate, the more stimulating chemical (theobromine) it contains.

Cocoa butter fats trigger natural endorphins and tiny amounts of anandamide, to create a "happiness high." And research shows that regular dark chocolate eaters are slimmer than those who abstain altogether.

Dates

Rich, sweet, and full of fiber, magnesium, potassium, and health-promoting polyphenols, dates are my ideal postworkout snack. The most common varieties are the meltingly soft, plump Medjool date and the firmer Deglet Noor date. Try topping a few with a sliced-up banana half and a tablespoon of nut butter.

Edamame (Whole Soybeans)

Eating edamame boosts your fiber and protein intake while lowering your saturated fats. Soybeans are an easy stand-in for chips, snack-worthy but not bad for your diet. A study in the *Journal of the American Medical Association* showed that a diet of soy protein, fiber from oats and barley, almonds, and margarine from plant sterols lowered cholesterol as much as statins, the most widely prescribed cholesterol medicine.

Eggs

Small but mighty, eggs make every calorie count by delivering more biologically usable protein than any other food—even beef. And don't de-yolk your omelet completely; in addition to protein, the yolk contains vitamin B_{12}, necessary for fat breakdown and muscle contraction. Eggs are packed with riboflavin, folate, and vitamins B_6, B_{12}, D, and E, as well as iron, phosphorus, selenium, zinc, and omega-3s.

Extra-Firm Tofu

This superversatile meatless option is easy to cook with and provides all the benefits meat brings to the table. A 6-ounce serving contains 24 grams of protein in less than 200 calories.

Garlic, Onions, Chives, Shallots

You may skip these ingredients before a date, but any other time I highly recommend incorporating them into your meals. The sulfur compounds found in these breath-busting superspices aren't just associated with warding off vampires—they're also linked with preventing colon, breast, and lung cancers. Epidemiological studies show that people who consume the most garlic and onions have a lower risk of stomach, colorectal, and prostate cancers. The active compounds in garlic are released when you crush the cloves, and they become more robust when sautéed in a little olive oil.

Grapes

Besides providing protection from heart attack and stroke, antioxidants in red grapes may also help keep your skin flexible and elastic. Researchers from the University of California also linked resveratrol, a chemical in grapes' skin, with preventing colon cancer.

Green Tea

Studies show that green tea—infused with the powerful catechin EGCG (epigallocatechin gallate)—reduces the risk of most types of cancer. The phytonutrients in the tea also support the growth of healthy intestinal bacteria. Some studies have found green tea extract to be useful for obesity management since it induces thermogenesis and stimulates fat oxidation. And EGCG is said to increase resting metabolism and stimulate fat-burning.

Hot Chile Peppers

Poblanos, serranos, habaneros, and jalapeños—all variations of chile peppers contain compounds called capsaicinoids, which give them their spicy heat. They are high in carotene and flavonoids and contain more than twice the amount of vitamin C found in citrus fruits.

Hummus

Remember our talk about chickpeas (see Beans and Legumes on page 194)? Well, mash 'em up with some tahini or buy premade hummus and you'll reap all the protein-rich goodness, not to mention fiber, of chickpeas in a delicious dip or spread. Adding tahini (ground sesame seeds) will deliver a tasty dose of omega-3 fatty acids and won't cost you more than 100 calories per 2-tablespoon serving.

Low-Fat Dressing

A little fat can do your body good, according to researchers from Purdue University. A study published in *Molecular Nutrition & Food Research* shows that eating monounsaturated fat can dramatically improve how many nutrients we absorb from food. Without a little fat in our salads, we can't reap all the good stuff from lettuce, carrots, tomatoes, and other healthy toppings. So swerve from the fat-free options and use a low-fat dressing instead (researchers recommend varieties with 3 grams of monounsaturated fat). Or try adding avocados, nuts, and olives to your salad to savor the same kind of monounsaturated fats found in dressing.

Low-Fat Milk

We tend to stray from dairy as we get older, but the benefits of a tall glass of calcium- and protein-rich goodness don't expire with age. Another beautiful thing about milk is that it has substance, so it helps you feel satisfied quickly and forestalls bingeing—just make sure you're not dunking any cookies in it. A University of Tennessee study reported dieters who consumed 1,200 to 1,300 milligrams of calcium-rich foods a day lost nearly twice as much weight as those taking in less calcium. During times of heavy training, I need to eat before going to the gym in order to keep my blood sugar stable and supply my muscles with a steady stream of protein so I reach for milk. Also, one of my favorite snacks right before bed is warm low-fat milk. It has a great combination of protein, fat, and carbs in the form of milk sugars!

Nuts and Nut Butters

Numerous studies give nuts an A+ for nutritious snacking because they are one of the best sources for heart-healthy monounsaturated fats, minerals, and fiber. In a study of more than 3,000 African American men and women, those who ate nuts at least five times a week cut their risk of dying of heart disease by 44 percent compared with people who ate nuts less frequently. Just be sure to keep track of your portion size (limit it to ¼ cup, or about a handful), as mindless popping will add up the calories. Also aim to incorporate these varieties: almonds, Brazil nuts, hazelnuts, macadamia nuts, pistachios, pecans, peanuts (actually a legume), and walnuts. Walnuts are worth a second look. A new study published in the *Journal of Nutrition* found that eating walnuts regularly could reduce your risk of developing type 2 diabetes. Researchers analyzed data collected by the Nurses' Health Studies, two decade-long studies that tracked the diets and health records of 138,000 women. While all of the participants were disease free at the beginning of the study, 5,930 developed type 2 diabetes during the 10-year span. Women who ate at least 8 ounces of walnuts a month (that's a little more than 2 cups of walnut halves) had a 24 percent lower risk of developing the disease than women who rarely ate walnuts. And the walnut eaters were also leaner than the women who ate nuts only on occasion.

Oatmeal

It's the foundation on which a nutritious breakfast is built—it's warm, filling, and digests slowly so you get long-lasting energy to keep you going all morning long without weighing you down. Oatmeal is also rich in soluble fiber, noted for its ability to reduce cholesterol. You may be tempted to try the instant varieties, but beware: These are often gooey and contain heaping amounts of sugar. Try unflavored varieties and sweeten them with berries, raisins, milk, or a touch of agave nectar.

Oils

A slew of oils support dieting and health. Here are some of my faves.

Avocado oil: The monounsaturated fats in this silky fruit oil help combat joint pain and promote soft skin. You can incorporate this natural painkiller in your daily diet (just mix it with a touch of soybean oil).

Coconut oil: The star power of coconuts comes from their lauric acid and healthy saturated fats, called medium-chain triglycerides. Research has linked this antioxidant-rich uberoil with balancing cholesterol levels, improving digestion, and reducing belly fat.

Olive oil: It may have a wimpy name, but it's a powerhouse in curbing cravings, burning fat, and building lean muscle. The monounsaturated fats found in it are tied to reducing risk of heart disease and osteoporosis and preventing muscle breakdown by lowering levels of cellular proteins linked to muscle wasting and weakness. Go for extra virgin varieties, which have higher levels of vitamin E.

Sesame oil: Its antioxidants, coupled with compounds called lignans, may help control blood sugar, thwart cavities, and lower LDL (bad) cholesterol, and it can even be used topically to prevent sunburn.

Walnut oil: You know you need omega-3s, but you can't stand fishy foods or capsules? Try this instead. Walnut oil is rich in fatty acids and contains alpha-linolenic acid, which serves as a building block for healthy fats that help regulate your immune and nervous system. What's more, research shows this oil can keep your stress levels and blood pressure in check to protect your ticker.

Pork Chops

Trim down to lean meat to get your protein. Researchers reported pork helped people preserve their muscle while still losing weight. Pork chops contain five times the selenium—a mineral linked to lowering risk of certain cancers—of beef and twice that of chicken. Stick with a 6-ounce serving.

Protein Powders and Bars

I'm a big fan of specialty foods like protein powders and protein bars because they are very convenient options for quick protein and on-the-go fuel. I like to construct my own protein shakes and smoothies, so I prefer to choose protein-only powders instead of using ready-made meal replacement shakes. I lean toward whey protein isolate, casein, and some vegan powders. My go-to brands are Tera's Whey and Vega, but there are dozens of good types to choose from. Protein powders are brilliant to consume before and after workouts because they deliver fast-digesting protein to your muscles when they most need it. Combining the protein with a fast-digesting carbohydrate like agave nectar or bananas helps to speed the delivery of protein to the muscles after a workout. I also use protein bars around my workouts if I am running late and don't have time to make a protein shake. I like Promax protein bars because they have four different formulations based on different workout needs. For example, there are bars made for fueling longer, harder kinds of workouts that demand different nutrition than recovery-type workouts.

Quinoa

This nutty-tasting grain has about twice the protein of regular cereal grains, fewer carbohydrates, and even some healthful fats. It's considered a complete protein, like eggs, because it contains all of the essential amino acids your body needs for muscle growth. And while quinoa and brown rice are on par calorie-wise, quinoa contains about 6 percent more fiber, 3 grams more protein, and higher amounts of potassium and iron. Try to get quinoa into your weekly meal plan, using it as a substitute for brown rice or sweet potatoes. You'll find it in the health food section of your supermarket. Quinoa can be used for making pilafs, risottos, salads, and soups, or even as a breakfast cereal with a sprinkling of cinnamon. If you haven't tried it yet, give this quick quinoa salad recipe a shot: Boil 1 cup of quinoa in a mixture of 1 cup pear juice and 1 cup water. Let cool. In a large bowl, toss with 2 diced apples, 1 cup fresh blueberries, $\frac{1}{2}$ cup chopped walnuts, and 1 cup plain yogurt. You'll love it.

Sardines

Okay, so the can may be a little creepy, but there's nothing fishy about the high amounts of omega-3 fatty acid and protein packed into each container of sardines. Fish oil is an anti-inflammatory agent that also protects against heart arrhythmias. A single can of sardines has more calcium than a cup of whole milk. Still not sold? Try chopping them up and tossing them into a salad. I promise the omega-3s are worth it—these fatty acids help suppress the activity of prostaglandins and leukotrienes, which can activate various diseases, cause blood clots, and inflame joints. I learned to love sardines after I discovered how incredibly healthful they are. Now I enjoy eating them on crunchy crackers with gourmet mustard.

Seeds

Flaxseeds: These are one of the few plant sources of healthful omega-3 fatty acids. But be sure to buy ground flaxseeds, or grind them yourself—whole seeds can pass through you undigested. Toss them into your oatmeal, protein shakes, yogurt, soups, and stews—or try them as an ice cream topping to balance out your periodic indulgences.

Pumpkin seeds: The pumpkin spice latte may be a staple of the fall season, but there aren't many bennies in the bottom of an empty latte cup. Swap the sugary beverages for seeds to get your pumpkin fix. Pumpkin seeds supply your body with a boost of magnesium, a mineral with a ton of perks. Increasing your body's magnesium intake has been associated with improved digestion and circulation and with pain relief.

Spinach

Popeye's favorite food wasn't just helping his muscles. Spinach and other iron-rich leafy green vegetables are also associated with helping women retain memory as they age, according to a recent study from Harvard University. Stuck on how to get over your inner child's rebellion against leafy greens? Try baking baby spinach with a dash of olive oil and sea salt. You'll reap all the bennies and still satisfy your cravings for crunch.

Sweet Potatoes

These are higher in fiber and lower in carbohydrates than white potatoes. Here's another reason to love them: They may help you look younger. European researchers recently found that pigments from beta-carotene-rich foods like sweet potatoes and carrots build up in your skin, helping to prevent ultraviolet rays from prematurely aging skin cells.

Tomatoes

According to the FDA, eating tomatoes may reduce the risk of gastric and pancreatic cancers thanks to their high concentration of lycopene, a carotenoid antioxidant. You don't have to eat fresh ones either to reap these benefits: Spaghetti and pizza sauces deliver them, too, since cooking doesn't reduce lycopene's potency.

Tropical Fruit

Kiwifruit: These small, odd-looking fruits are loaded with vitamin C and fiber.

Oranges: You know oranges are the big man on campus when it comes to supplying vitamin C, but they also contain anti-inflammatory compounds called flavonoids that may help repair DNA and prevent cancer growth.

Papayas: If you have a cold, eat a papaya. One medium papaya delivers more than 300 percent of the recommended amount of vitamin C (take that, orange!). The beta-carotene and vitamins C and E in papayas reduce inflammation throughout the body, aiding your immune system.

Turkey

This deli counter favorite is a great option for sandwiches, or try dried turkey as a portable snack. Six thin slices of whole cut, lean turkey can power you up with 10 grams of protein for just 50 calories! Subbing in turkey jerky for regular beef jerky is easier on your digestive system while still supplying ample amounts of protein to keep your muscles happy.

Whole Grain Cereal

I'll always be an egg advocate. But when you're sick of scrambled eggs and need a quick fix, Kashi GoLean or Honey Sunshine cereal is the breakfast of champions. GoLean is made with Kashi's trademark "seven whole grains," which bring you 13 grams of protein and 10 grams of fiber in fewer than 250 calories. British researchers recently found that people who eat a carbohydrate-rich, high-fiber breakfast before working out burn twice as much fat as they do after a similar meal without all the roughage. If you're converting from sugared cereal to healthier choices, try Kashi's Honey Sunshine for a natural jolt of sugar.

Whole Wheat Bread and Pasta

The main difference between white and whole wheat anything can be found in the processing. Whole wheat contains three parts of the grain: bran, germ, and endosperm. White bread is stripped of the bran and germ in processing. While endosperm still packs iron and, of course, a decent serving of carbohydrates, you don't want to skip the benefits of the full trio. Whole grain varieties contain vitamin E, B vitamins, antioxidants, fiber, protein, and even a little healthy fat. Since

Enjoy a Leaner Pizza

How you order your pie can make the difference, adding or subtracting hundreds of calories. Try these calorie-cutting tips.

1. **Know what a topping will get you.** Choosing spinach, green peppers, roasted peppers, mushrooms, or onions will add fewer than 5 calories per slice. Here's what you'll save per slice by avoiding these meaty options.

   Pepperoni: 30 calories
   Bacon: 43 calories
   Italian sausage: 44 calories
   Ground beef: 38 calories
   Chicken: 18 calories
   Ham: 11 calories

2. **Cut the cheese.** Ask the pizza baker to make your pie with half the usual amount of cheese. Savings per slice: 85 calories.

3. **Order thin crust.** You'll save 49 calories per slice over regular pizza.

4. **Try a tomato pie.** Sauce-only pizzas are delicious with a tablespoon of grated Parmesan cheese. Savings per slice: 63 calories.

400 Calories Gone!

Four hundred calories is a significant number to cut out of your daily diet, but it's actually pretty easy to do if you make some smart swaps. Here are a handful of ways to save without sacrifice.

- Avoid the calorie-dense cocktails like the piña colada (two drinks deliver 656 calories) and drink two 6-ounce glasses of red wine instead (300 calories). Keep your hand out of the bowl of bar nuts (44 calories per scoop) and you'll have saved 400 calories.

- Cut up a large apple (116 calories), top it with 1 cup of plain yogurt (149 calories), and sprinkle a teaspoon of cinnamon (6 calories) on top. Choose this dessert over a piece of apple pie (411 calories) with a cup of vanilla ice cream (274 calories). Savings: 414 calories.

- Instead of the Cheddar (113 calories per slice) and egg on a bagel (360 calories), breakfast on eggs with a slice of whole wheat toast (75 calories). Savings: 398 calories.

- Make your breakfast to-go. Have a granola bar (118 calories) instead of a bowl of granola (299 calories) with 1 cup of whole milk (149 calories). Eat a medium navel orange (60 calories) instead of drinking 10 ounces of processed orange juice (150 calories). Savings: 420 calories.

- Save money and calories by skipping the smoothie made at the franchise store. Make your own: Blend 2 slices of pineapple, 1 apple, 1 peeled beet, 1 carrot, ½ cup organic apple juice, and a dash of water and ice. One serving is only 115 calories. Save the second for an evening snack. Savings: 485 calories.

- Substitute 2 cups of spaghetti squash (84 calories) for 2 cups of pasta (443 calories) and top it with 1 cup of tomato sauce. Season it with freshly ground black pepper instead of 2 tablespoons of shredded Parmesan cheese (44 calories). Savings: 403 calories.

Food Fact

On average, women who read nutrition labels weigh 9 pounds less than women who don't.

Source: *Agricultural Economics*

the whole grain is tougher to break down (unlike enriched white bread), you'll feel fuller longer and be able to reap the slow-digesting benefits of all the above.

Wild Salmon

This fish is rich in the omega-3 fatty acid DHA (docosahexaenoic acid). People with the highest blood levels of this nutrient have a 47 percent lower chance of developing dementia, according to a study published in the *Archives of Neurology*. DHA, a component of neurons, plays a key role in memory and learning. It's best to eat wild salmon rather than farmed fish; farmed salmon may not get the appropriate marine diet needed to produce high amounts of omega-3s.

Yogurt

In an *International Journal of Obesity* study, dieters who had three servings of yogurt a day for 12 weeks lost more fat around their waists than a control group. Yogurt also has probiotics, healthy bacteria that may help reduce bloating if eaten regularly. You can find probiotics in kefir, a yogurtlike milk product, and in supplements, too.

The probiotics naturally found in yogurt aren't just good for your gut. Live cultures, such as those found in Greek yogurt, are also associated with boosting your brainpower, according to research published in the journal *Gastroenterology*. Greek yogurt has a thicker texture than traditional yogurts, not to mention twice as much protein. Avoid fat-free versions that tend to hide harmful artificial sweeteners, and instead opt for a full-fat version. Sweeten lightly with $\frac{1}{2}$ tablespoon of agave, or embrace the versatility of plain yogurt and try it as a substitute for sour cream.

Chapter 16
Lift to Get Lean Recipes

A lot of women overlook one of the hidden gems in strength training. It's a welcome side benefit of all the effort you put into your workouts: You get to eat more, much more, and satisfying food, too. Remember, the more muscle you carry, the more calories you burn even when you aren't doing three sets of Lunges. That means extra food won't go to your bottom or your belly. So eat, ladies! It is important to fuel your workouts for energy and strength. Here are some favorite recipes to help you do just that using many of the powerful ingredients we discussed in the last chapter.

Breakfasts
Asparagus with Eggs and Parmesan

1   **bunch asparagus**
4   **large eggs**
       Ground black pepper
2   **tablespoons shaved Parmesan cheese**

1. Preheat the oven to 425°F. In an oiled 11″ x 7″ baking dish, spread the asparagus. Bake for 15 minutes, or until crisp-tender.
2. Crack the eggs over the top and sprinkle with the pepper. Bake for 10 minutes, or until the whites are set and the yolks reach desired doneness.
3. Top with the Parmesan cheese.

Makes 4 servings

Per serving: 94 calories, 9 g protein, 3 g carbohydrates, 6 g total fat (2 g saturated fat), 1 g fiber, 109 mg sodium

Date-Oatmeal Stuffed Apples

½   cup cold cooked oatmeal
¼   cup chopped toasted hazelnuts
5   dates, pitted and chopped
1   tablespoon maple syrup
¼   teaspoon ground nutmeg
     Pinch of salt
4   Rome apples
½   cup apple juice
4   teaspoons vanilla Greek yogurt

1. Preheat the oven to 375°F. In a medium bowl, mix together the oatmeal, hazelnuts, dates, maple syrup, nutmeg, and salt.

2. Use a melon baller to make a cavity three-quarters deep in each of the apples. Pack the cavities with the filling.

3. Place the apples in a 24" x 18" baking dish. Pour the apple juice around them, cover with foil, and bake for 40 minutes to 1 hour 10 minutes, until tender.

4. Top each apple with 1 teaspoon of Greek yogurt.

Makes 4 servings

Per serving: 269 calories, 3 g protein, 58 g carbohydrates, 6 g total fat (1 g saturated fat), 8 g fiber, 41 mg sodium

Eggs Benedict

1   Thomas' 100% Whole Wheat English Muffin
1   apple, halved and cored
    Splash of white wine vinegar
2   eggs
2   tablespoons fat-free plain Greek yogurt
$\frac{1}{4}$ teaspoon dried dill
$\frac{1}{4}$ teaspoon lemon juice
$\frac{1}{2}$ teaspoon grated lemon peel
2   sprigs fresh dill

1. Lightly toast the English muffin.

2. Slice the apple halves into $\frac{1}{2}$" cross sections.

3. Fill a medium pan with about 5" of water. Bring the water to a low boil. Add the vinegar and swirl the pan until it is evenly distributed. Break an egg into a cup and pour it slowly into the water, with the white entering first. Allow the egg white to set around the yolk like a white pillow. When poached, the yolk will float to the top. Use a spoon to remove and place on a paper towel to absorb excess water. Do the same with the second egg.

4. In a small bowl, combine the yogurt, dried dill, lemon juice, and lemon peel. Whisk until smooth.

5. On the first half of the English muffin, stack half the apple slices, then an egg. Drizzle with half of the yogurt sauce and top with a sprig of fresh dill. Repeat with the second half of the English muffin to create 2 open-faced sandwiches.

Makes 1 serving

Per serving: 370 calories, 21 g protein, 50 g carbohydrates, 12 g total fat (3 g saturated fat), 8 g fiber, 618 mg sodium

Egg 'n' Greens

1	tablespoon olive oil, divided
1	cup sliced mushrooms
2	cups spinach
1	egg
1	tablespoon Sriracha sauce

1. In a large skillet over medium heat, warm half the oil. Cook the mushrooms and spinach, stirring frequently, until the mushrooms are lightly browned. Remove to a plate.

2. Add the remaining oil to the skillet.

3. Crack the egg into the pan and cook it sunny-side-up.

4. Add the egg to the vegetables. Drizzle with the Sriracha.

Makes 1 serving

Per serving: 216 calories, 10 g protein, 4 g carbohydrates, 19 g total fat (4 g saturated fat), 2 g fiber, 476 mg sodium

Brown Rice Bowl

Splash of white wine vinegar

1   **egg**

²⁄₃   **cup cooked brown rice**

½   **cooked sweet potato, sliced**

1   **cooked beet, sliced**

¼   **cup chopped cooked acorn squash**

1. First, poach the egg. Fill a medium pan with about 5″ of water. Bring the water to a low boil. Add the vinegar and swirl the pan until it is evenly distributed. Break the egg into a cup and pour it slowly into the water, with the white entering first. Allow the egg white to set around the yolk like a white pillow. When poached, the egg will float to the top. Use a spoon to remove it and place it on a paper towel to absorb excess water.

2. In a bowl, combine the rice, sweet potato, beet, and squash.

3. Top with the poached egg.

Makes 1 serving

Per serving: 318 calories, 12 g protein, 54 g carbohydrates, 6 g total fat (2 g saturated fat), 7 g fiber, 235 mg sodium

Power Breakfast

2	slices whole grain bread
2	teaspoons low-sodium honey mustard
½	tomato, thinly sliced
½	avocado, sliced
1	teaspoon olive oil
2	fresh basil leaves
	Fresh ground pepper to taste
½	tablespoon ground flaxseeds

1. Toast the bread slices.

2. Spread the honey mustard on both slices.

3. Place the tomato and avocado on 1 slice of bread, topping them with the olive oil, basil, pepper, and flaxseeds.

4. Top with the other slice of bread to create a sandwich.

5. Cut into quarters for an easier on-the-go meal!

Makes 1 serving

Per serving: 597 calories, 29 g protein, 79 g carbohydrates, 20 g total fat (5 g saturated fat), 11 g fiber, 209 mg sodium

Pumped-Up Banana-Pecan Oatmeal

¼   cup quick-cooking Irish oatmeal

½   cup water

½   scoop vanilla whey protein powder

1   teaspoon ground cinnamon

⅛   teaspoon salt

¼   cup fat-free milk

1   banana, sliced

1   tablespoon pecan pieces

1. In a microwaveable bowl, whip together the oatmeal, water, protein powder, cinnamon, and salt.

2. Microwave the mixture on high for 90 seconds.

3. Top with the milk, banana, and pecan pieces.

Makes 1 serving

Per serving: 389 calories, 18 g protein, 63 g carbohydrates, 9 g total fat (2 g saturated fat), 9 g fiber, 349 mg sodium

Stuffed Cinnamon French Toast

2   tablespoons part-skim ricotta cheese
2   slices whole wheat bread
1   teaspoon honey
      Pinch + ½ teaspoon ground cinnamon
½   tablespoon sliced almonds
1   egg
1   tablespoon fat-free milk
      Handful of fresh berries
      Confectioners' sugar (optional)

1. Spread the ricotta on 1 slice of bread.

2. Drizzle with the honey and sprinkle with a pinch of cinnamon.

3. Top with the sliced almonds and the other slice of bread.

4. In a medium bowl, whisk together the egg, milk, and ½ teaspoon cinnamon.

5. Coat the sandwich in the egg mixture and cook it on a nonstick griddle over medium heat, turning once, until the bread is lightly browned on both sides and the cheese is melted.

6. Serve with the berries. Sprinkle with confectioners' sugar, if desired.

Makes 1 serving

Per serving: 337 calories, 19 g protein, 50 g carbohydrates, 12 g total fat (4 g saturated fat), 8 g fiber, 335 mg sodium

Sweet and Spicy Quinoa Hash

1	teaspoon coconut oil
	Pinch of red-pepper flakes
½	cup cubed sweet potato
⅓	cup chopped kale
1	clove garlic, minced
	Pinch of salt
½	cup cooked quinoa

1. In a skillet over medium heat, warm the coconut oil.

2. Add the red-pepper flakes and sweet potato.

3. Cook, stirring frequently, for about 5 minutes.

4. Stir in the kale, garlic, and salt. Cook, stirring frequently, for 3 minutes longer or until the kale has wilted.

5. Add the quinoa and heat through.

Makes 1 serving

Per serving: 426 calories, 14 g protein, 71 g carbohydrates, 10 g total fat (5 g saturated fat), 9 g fiber, 206 mg sodium

Tofu Scramble

1	teaspoon olive oil
4	ounces soft tofu, crumbled
½	large red bell pepper, chopped
⅔	cup chopped baby portobello mushrooms
1	cup chopped spinach
1	Arnold Sandwich Thins 100% Whole Wheat
¼	cup (1 ounce) shredded part-skim mozzarella
½	teaspoon dried oregano

1. Heat the oil in a skillet over medium-high heat. Add the tofu, red pepper, mushrooms, and spinach. Cook for 5 to 7 minutes, stirring frequently.

2. Serve the tofu scramble on the sandwich thin.

3. Top with the cheese and oregano.

Makes 1 serving

Per serving: 333 calories, 22 g protein, 28 g carbohydrates, 15 g total fat (4 g saturated fat), 7 g fiber, 360 mg sodium

Lunches
Asian Edamame Salad

SALAD

1	head red cabbage, shredded
1	cup steamed, shelled edamame
4	carrots, cut into matchsticks
1	red bell pepper, cut into matchsticks
½	cup chopped fresh cilantro

GINGER-MISO DRESSING

1	piece ginger (2"), finely chopped
1	clove garlic, minced
2	tablespoons white miso
2	tablespoons sesame oil
½	cup rice wine vinegar
1	tablespoon agave nectar

1. **To make the salad:** In a large bowl, combine the cabbage, edamame, carrots, bell pepper, and cilantro.

2. **To make the dressing:** In a medium bowl, whisk together the ginger, garlic, miso, sesame oil, vinegar, and agave nectar. Add to the salad and toss to coat.

Makes 4 servings

Per serving: 220 calories, 8 g protein, 29 g carbohydrates, 9 g total fat (1 g saturated fat), 9 g fiber, 410 mg sodium

TOP IT OFF

To liven up your salad, try any of these tasty, nutritious add-ons.

Hemp Hearts. Shelled hemp seeds are one of the densest sources of plant protein and an excellent source of iron, magnesium, and both omega-3 and omega-6 fatty acids.

Fennel. Thinly sliced fennel bulb provides a refreshing crunch and can also aid digestion.

Sauerkraut (or Kimchi). Fermented foods filled with probiotic goodness, sauerkraut and kimchi are low in calories and lend tanginess and spice.

Quinoa. Bulk up your salad with this high-protein favorite—it cooks in just 15 minutes on the stove.

Blueberries. Packed with antioxidants, blueberries are bursting with flavor and have only 10 calories per ½ cup.

Beef and Veggie Salad Bowl

2	tablespoons dry red quinoa
2	cups mesclun greens
3	ounces cooked lean beef, cubed
½	cup chopped broccoli florets
¼	red bell pepper, chopped
2	teaspoons olive oil
1	teaspoon red wine vinegar

1. Cook the quinoa according to package directions.

2. In a medium bowl, toss the quinoa with the greens, beef, broccoli, and red pepper.

3. In a small bowl, whisk together the oil and vinegar to make a dressing. Add the dressing to the salad, toss to coat, and serve.

Makes 1 serving

Per serving: 353 calories, 31 g protein, 21 g carbohydrates, 17 g total fat (4 g saturated fat), 5 g fiber, 138 mg sodium

Bison Burgers

12	**ounces ground grass-fed bison**
½	**cup chopped onion**
½	**teaspoon garlic powder**
¼	**teaspoon smoked paprika**

1. Coat a grill rack or broiler-pan rack with cooking spray. Preheat the grill or broiler.
2. In a medium bowl, mix together the bison, onion, garlic powder, and paprika.
3. Form the mixture into 4 patties.
4. Grill for 5 to 6 minutes, then flip and grill for another 5 to 6 minutes, or until the burgers reach an internal temperature of 155°F.

Makes 4 servings

Per serving: 230 calories, 19 g protein, 11 g carbohydrates, 14 g total fat (4 g saturated fat), 5 g fiber, 227 mg sodium

Fix 'n' Eat Sardine Sandy

1   can (3.75 ounces) low-sodium sardines packed in water, drained, rinsed, and patted dry

2   slices Ezekiel 4:9 Organic Sprouted 100% Whole Grain Flourless Low Sodium Bread

     Low-sodium honey mustard

1. Lay the sardines on 1 slice of bread.
2. Add the honey mustard (to taste).
3. Top with the other slice of bread.

Makes 1 serving

Per serving: 370 calories, 22 g protein, 31 g carbohydrates, 18 g total fat (8 g saturated fat), 7 g fiber, 4 mg sodium

Salmon-Avocado "Sushi"

½   avocado, thinly sliced
2   ounces smoked salmon, thinly sliced
¼   cup cooked rice noodles
¼   papaya, thinly sliced
1   tablespoon chopped scallions
2   sheets nori seaweed
1   lime wedge
     Salt and ground black pepper

1.   Lay half the avocado, salmon, noodles, papaya, and scallions on each nori sheet.

2.   Roll up the nori sheets with the ingredients inside, sushi-style.

3.   Cut into 1" pieces.

4.   Squeeze the lime wedge over the "sushi," and sprinkle it with salt and pepper to taste.

Makes 1 serving

Per serving: 395 calories, 37 g protein, 26 g carbohydrates, 17 g total fat (3 g saturated fat), 7 g fiber, 207 mg sodium

Tofu Salad

1	tablespoon soy sauce
1	tablespoon almond butter
$\frac{1}{8}$	teaspoon minced garlic
4	ounces extra-firm tofu, thinly sliced
1	cup slivered snow peas
$\frac{1}{2}$	teaspoon sesame seeds
2	Scandinavian crispbread crackers

1. In a medium bowl, whisk together the soy sauce, almond butter, and garlic.

2. Add the tofu and snow peas and toss to coat.

3. Top with the sesame seeds.

4. Serve with the crackers.

Makes 1 serving

Per serving: 241 calories, 14 g protein, 21 g carbohydrates, 13 g total fat (2 g saturated fat), 5 g fiber, 1,090 mg sodium

Turkey and Avocado Sandwich with Slaw

SANDWICH

1   tablespoon brown mustard
2   slices rye bread
3   ounces low-sodium skinless turkey breast
2   slices tomato
1   slice red onion
¼   cup sliced avocado

SLAW

2   tablespoons golden raisins
1   cup shredded green cabbage
1   cup shredded red cabbage

1. **To make the sandwich:** Spread the mustard on 1 slice of bread. Stack the turkey, tomato, onion, and avocado on the bread. Top with the other bread slice.

2. **To make the slaw:** In a medium bowl, combine the raisins and cabbage.

3. Serve together.

Makes 1 serving

Per serving: 495 calories, 29 g protein, 69 g carbohydrates, 14 g total fat (2 g saturated fat), 14 g fiber, 1,270 mg sodium

Turkey-Orange Salad

½   **navel orange, cut into small chunks**
2   **teaspoons extra virgin olive oil**
     Salt and ground black pepper
1   **cup packed mixed salad greens**
⅓   **cup (2 ounces) skinless roast turkey chunks**
2   **thin slices red onion, quartered**

1. Place the orange in a mixing bowl. Add the oil and salt and pepper to taste. Toss with a fork, pressing a few orange chunks lightly to release their juice.

2. Add the greens, turkey, and onion. Toss with the orange dressing to coat.

3. Transfer the salad to a serving plate.

Makes 1 serving

Per serving: 224 calories, 19 g protein, 12 g carbohydrates, 11 g total fat (2 g saturated fat), 3 g fiber, 52 mg sodium

Dinners
Asian Salmon

1	tablespoon extra virgin olive oil
	Grated peel of 1 lime
2	tablespoons ground coriander
1	teaspoon finely chopped fresh ginger
4	pieces (4 ounces each) wild salmon
2	tablespoons honey
¼	teaspoon ground black pepper
2	tablespoons gluten-free light soy sauce

1. Preheat the oven to 225°F. In a small bowl, combine the oil, lime peel, coriander, and ginger.

2. Place the salmon in an ovenproof baking dish and brush it with the oil mixture.

3. Bake the salmon for 15 minutes, then turn on the broiler and crisp it for 3 more minutes.

4. While the salmon is baking, in a small bowl, mix the honey and black pepper. To serve, drizzle the honey mixture and soy sauce over the fish.

Makes 4 servings

Per serving: 320 calories, 24 g protein, 11 g carbohydrates, 19 g total fat (4 g saturated fat), 1 g fiber, 330 mg sodium

Cod Cakes

Try making these crisp and devilishly good patties using any fish you like. You can also use canned or leftover fish instead of starting from scratch. Just sub in 2 large cans of salmon or tuna, drained, or 2 cups of flaked cooked fish for the cod.

1	pound cod, cut into large chunks
½	teaspoon salt, divided
¼	cup + 2 tablespoons 2% plain Greek yogurt
¼	cup chopped parsley
1	egg yolk, beaten
1	tablespoon Dijon mustard
1	tablespoon freshly squeezed lemon juice (from ½ lemon)
6	tablespoons + ½ cup panko bread crumbs
3	scallions, minced
¼	teaspoon freshly ground black pepper
¼	cup canola oil

1. Put about an inch of water in the bottom of a large nonstick skillet and bring it to a simmer over medium-high heat. Season the fish with ¼ teaspoon of the salt and add the fish to the pan. Cover the pan and simmer over low heat until the fish flakes easily, about 6 to 8 minutes. Remove the fish from the pan with a slotted spoon and drain it on paper towels. Pour out the water and dry the skillet. Allow the fish to cool slightly, about 5 minutes, and pat it completely dry.

2. In a medium bowl, using 2 forks or your fingers, flake the fish by breaking it apart and removing any bones. Add the yogurt, parsley, egg yolk, mustard, lemon juice, 6 tablespoons of the panko, scallions, pepper, and remaining ¼ teaspoon salt. Stir to combine.

(continued)

3. Shape the mixture into 8 round cakes. Coat the cakes with the remaining $\frac{1}{2}$ cup panko and pat off the excess.

4. Heat 2 tablespoons of the oil in the nonstick skillet over medium heat. Add the cakes and cook for 2 to 3 minutes, or until brown and crisp on the bottom. Add the remaining 2 tablespoons oil, turn the cakes, and cook until golden brown on the other side, about 2 to 3 minutes longer.

5. Drain on paper towels. Serve hot.

Makes 4 servings

Per serving: 211 calories, 20 g protein, 6 g carbohydrates, 11 g total fat (2 g saturated fat), 1 g fiber, 307 mg sodium

Beef and Asparagus Salad

ROAST BEEF

2   pounds center cut beef tenderloin

½   teaspoon sea salt

1   teaspoon ground black pepper

SALAD

8   cups water

2   pounds asparagus, trimmed

2   tablespoons chopped fresh basil

2   tablespoons grated lemon peel

2   tablespoons fresh lemon juice

½   teaspoon sea salt

CAPER OIL

2   tablespoons + 1 teaspoon olive oil

1   teaspoon capers, drained and rinsed

1. **To make the roast beef:** Preheat the oven to 350°F. Season the beef with the sea salt and pepper. Heat a large skillet over high heat. Sear the beef until light brown, about 5 minutes. Place the roast in a 24" x 18" baking pan and insert a meat thermometer into the center. Roast for 45 minutes, or until the internal temperature reaches 130°F. Remove from the oven and cool. Refrigerate for 2 hours.

2. **To make the salad:** Just before serving, bring the water to a boil in a large pot. Blanch the asparagus for 3 to 4 minutes, or until tender. Drain and place in ice water for 1 minute. Remove the asparagus and chop it into 1" pieces. In a large bowl, combine the asparagus, basil, lemon peel and juice, and sea salt. Mix well.

3. **To make the caper oil:** In a blender, puree the oil and capers.

4. **To serve:** Slice the beef thinly and serve 3 ounces with ½ cup of salad per person. Drizzle the beef with 1 teaspoon of the caper oil.

Makes 8 servings

Per serving: 287 calories, 35 g protein, 5 g carbohydrates, 13 g total fat (4 g saturated fat), 3 g fiber, 375 mg sodium

Chicken, Sweet Potato, and Apple Skillet

1   pound boneless, skinless chicken breasts, cut into $\frac{1}{2}$" cubes
      Salt
4   teaspoons olive oil, divided
3   slices 30% less fat center cut bacon, chopped
$1\frac{1}{2}$ cups trimmed and quartered Brussels sprouts
1   medium sweet potato, peeled and cut into $\frac{1}{2}$" cubes
1   medium onion, chopped
2   Golden Delicious apples, peeled, cored, and cut into $\frac{3}{4}$" cubes
4   cloves garlic, sliced
1   teaspoon chopped fresh thyme or $\frac{1}{4}$ teaspoon dried
$\frac{1}{4}$ teaspoon ground cinnamon
1   cup reduced-sodium chicken broth, divided
      Ground black pepper

1. Season the chicken lightly with salt.

2. Heat 2 teaspoons of the oil in a large nonstick or cast-iron skillet over medium-high heat. Add the chicken and cook until lightly browned and cooked through, about 5 minutes. Transfer to a plate.

3. Return the skillet to the heat and add the remaining 2 teaspoons oil. Stir in the bacon and cook for 2 minutes, or until starting to brown. Add the Brussels sprouts, sweet potato, and onion. Cook, stirring occasionally, until crisp-tender, about 5 minutes. Stir in the apples, garlic, thyme, and cinnamon. Cook for 3 minutes.

4. Pour in $\frac{1}{2}$ cup of the broth, bring to a boil, and cook 2 minutes longer, or until the broth has evaporated. Add the reserved chicken and remaining $\frac{1}{2}$ cup broth. Cook for 2 minutes, or until heated through. Season with the salt and black pepper as needed.

Makes 4 servings

Per serving: 309 calories, 29 g protein, 28 g carbohydrates, 10 g total fat (2 g saturated fat), 5 g fiber, 459 mg sodium

Turmeric Chicken with Apple-Shallot Confit

1	tablespoon finely chopped fresh turmeric root or 2 teaspoons ground
1	tablespoon olive oil
4	boneless, skinless chicken breast halves
	Salt
	Ground black pepper
1	cup finely chopped shallots
1	cup peeled and finely chopped apple
1	tablespoon sugar
2	tablespoons butter
1	tablespoon sherry vinegar

1. In a small bowl, combine the turmeric and oil. Rub the mixture on the chicken and season with salt and pepper to taste. Marinate for 2 hours.

2. In a medium saucepan, bring the shallots, apple, sugar, 1 teaspoon salt, and butter to a simmer over medium-low heat. Cook until browned, about 10 minutes. Add the vinegar and remove from the heat.

3. Coat a grill rack with cooking spray and preheat the grill. Grill the chicken for 3 to 5 minutes on each side, or until a thermometer inserted in the thickest portion registers 160°F and the juices run clear.

4. To serve, spoon ¼ cup of the caramelized apples and shallots over each chicken breast.

Makes 4 servings

Per serving: 320 calories, 36 g protein, 12 g carbohydrates, 13 g total fat (5 g saturated fat), 2 g fiber, 610 mg sodium

Tandoori Turkey Kebabs

1 cup fat-free plain yogurt

2 tablespoons garam masala

2½ teaspoons chopped jarred garlic

½ teaspoon ground ginger (optional)

Salt

1 pound turkey tenderloin, cut into 2" pieces

¾ cup dry whole wheat couscous

⅓ cup chopped dried fruit mix (any variety)

1. Soak 8 wooden skewers in a bowl of water and set aside.

2. Coat a grill rack with cooking spray and preheat the grill.

3. In a medium bowl, combine the yogurt, garam masala, garlic, ginger (if using), and salt to taste. Add the turkey and marinate for at least 10 minutes.

4. Meanwhile, prepare the couscous according to package instructions, adding the dried fruit during cooking.

5. Slide the turkey onto the skewers. Place the kebabs on the hot grill and cook, turning frequently, until the turkey is cooked through, about 10 to 12 minutes.

6. Place ½ cup couscous onto each of 4 plates.

7. Top each with 2 kebabs.

Makes 4 servings

Per serving: 283 calories, 34 g protein, 32 g carbohydrates, 3 g total fat (0 g saturated fat), 3 g fiber, 255 mg sodium

Quick Turkey-Spinach Lasagna

1¼ cups low-fat ricotta cheese

1 large egg

¼ teaspoon ground black pepper

1 tablespoon minced garlic

1 tablespoon dried oregano

1 can (28 ounces) organic crushed tomatoes

6 oven-ready lasagna noodles (half of a 12-ounce box)

3 cups finely chopped or torn baby spinach leaves

8 ounces skinless roast turkey, finely chopped

¾ cup shredded provolone cheese

1. Preheat the oven to 375°F. Lightly coat an 18" x 12" baking dish with cooking spray.

2. In a small bowl, beat the ricotta, egg, and pepper with a fork until well blended. Gently stir in the garlic and oregano.

3. Spread ¼ cup of the tomatoes over the bottom of the baking dish and place 3 noodles, overlapping slightly, over them.

4. Spread on half of the ricotta mixture, half of the spinach, half of the turkey, half of the remaining tomatoes, and half of the provolone.

5. Top with the remaining 3 noodles, ricotta mixture, spinach, turkey, tomatoes, and provolone.

6. Coat one side of a 14"-long piece of aluminum foil with cooking spray.

7. Lay the foil, sprayed side down, over the lasagna and loosely seal the edges.

8. Bake for 45 minutes, or until bubbling. Let sit for 5 minutes before serving.

Makes 6 servings

Per serving: 283 calories, 28 g protein, 28 g carbohydrates, 6 g total fat (3 g saturated fat), 4 g fiber, 613 mg sodium

Spinach Salad Pizza

Forget about ordering a side salad with your slice—you can just pile your greens right on top instead. This combo features blue cheese crumbles, which add a big kick of robust flavor for a fraction of the fat you'd get from a standard mozzarella-loaded piece of pizza. And best of all, there's zero cooking required.

1	cup baby spinach
½	cup sliced red grapes
1	teaspoon pine nuts
1	tablespoon blue cheese crumbles
1	tablespoon light balsamic vinaigrette
1	slice ready-made pizza crust

1. In a bowl, toss the spinach with the grapes, pine nuts, blue cheese crumbles, and light balsamic vinaigrette.
2. Top the slice of ready-made pizza crust with the salad.

Makes 1 serving

Per serving: 285 calories, 9 g protein, 51 g carbohydrates, 7 g total fat (2 g saturated fat), 3 g fiber, 670 mg sodium

Warm Chickpea-Quinoa Salad

1	cup dry quinoa or whole wheat couscous
	Vegetable broth
1½	teaspoons chopped garlic
1	small zucchini, quartered and sliced
2	carrots, grated
½	cup chopped red bell pepper
2	cups canned chickpeas, rinsed and drained
½	cup packed chopped scallions
2	tablespoons extra virgin olive oil
3	tablespoons white wine vinegar
¼	teaspoon salt
	Ground black pepper
4	cups fresh baby spinach leaves

1. Cook the quinoa or couscous according to package directions but use vegetable broth instead of water.

2. Coat a skillet with cooking spray and place it over medium-high heat. Add the garlic, zucchini, carrots, and bell pepper. Cook, stirring frequently, for 5 minutes or until softened. Add the chickpeas and continue cooking until heated through.

3. In a food processor, puree the scallions, gradually adding the oil, vinegar, salt, and black pepper to taste. Process to a thick consistency.

4. Add the scallion mixture and quinoa to the chickpea mixture and heat through.

5. To serve, arrange 1 cup spinach on each of 4 plates and pile equal amounts of the chickpea mixture on top.

Makes 4 servings

Per serving: 368 calories, 14 g protein, 54 g carbohydrates, 12 g total fat (1 g saturated fat), 11 g fiber, 353 mg sodium

Sides and Snacks
Asian Slaw

2   cups packaged broccoli slaw or regular slaw
⅓   cup finely chopped onion
½   cup shredded carrot
1   tablespoon chopped fresh cilantro
2   tablespoons chopped almonds
2   teaspoons toasted sesame oil
1½   tablespoons rice wine vinegar
¼   teaspoon red-pepper flakes

1.   In a bowl, mix the slaw, onion, carrot, cilantro, and almonds.
2.   In a separate bowl, mix the oil, vinegar, and pepper flakes.
3.   Pour the oil mixture over the vegetables and toss to coat.

Makes 2 servings

Per serving: 141 calories, 4 g protein, 13 g carbohydrates, 9 g total fat (1 g saturated fat), 5 g fiber, 44 mg sodium

Endive Leaves with Sardines, White Beans, and Orange

1	small orange
¼	cup rinsed, drained, and slightly mashed canned white beans
3	canned sardines packed in olive oil, halved or quartered and patted dry
4	pitted black olives, sliced
2	teaspoons extra virgin olive oil
	Sea salt and freshly ground black pepper
12	small endive leaves

1. Cut 12 small curls from the orange peel and reserve, wrapped in plastic.

2. Remove the rest of the peel and the white pith from the orange and, working over a bowl, release the orange segments from the membrane using a small, sharp knife, allowing both fruit and juices to fall into the bowl. Squeeze the membrane to extract any remaining juices.

3. Add the beans, sardines, olives, and oil to the bowl. Season to taste with sea salt and pepper and gently toss together.

4. Arrange the endive leaves on a platter and top them evenly with the orange mixture. Season with additional sea salt and pepper, if needed, and garnish with the reserved orange peel. Serve immediately.

Makes 12 servings

Per serving: 27 calories, 1 g protein, 3 g carbohydrates, 1 g total fat (0 g saturated fat), 1 g fiber, 26 mg sodium

Maple-Glazed Root Vegetables

1	pound small carrots, peeled, with 1″ of greens
½	pound small parsnips, peeled and quartered lengthwise
1	tablespoon extra virgin olive oil
⅛	teaspoon salt
⅛	teaspoon ground black pepper
1	tablespoon freshly grated ginger
1	clove garlic, minced
6	tablespoons pure maple syrup

1. Preheat the oven to 425°F. Lightly coat a rimmed baking sheet with cooking spray. In a large bowl, toss the carrots and parsnips with the oil and salt and pepper.

2. Spread the vegetables evenly on the baking sheet. Roast for 25 minutes, turning once, or until golden brown and tender.

3. During the last 5 minutes of roasting, set a small saucepan over medium heat. Add the ginger and garlic and cook until fragrant, about 1 minute. Add the maple syrup and stir to combine. Simmer until thick, about 2 to 3 minutes. Remove from the heat.

4. When the vegetables are done, transfer them to a serving dish and toss with the maple glaze.

Makes 4 servings

Per serving: 200 calories, 2 g protein, 42 g carbohydrates, 4 g total fat (0.5 g saturated fat), 6 g fiber, 300 mg sodium

Maple-Glazed Brussels Sprouts

1   **bag frozen Brussels sprouts, thawed**
2   **tablespoons maple syrup**
1   **tablespoon olive oil**
2   **teaspoons whole grain mustard**
      Salt

1. Pat the Brussels sprouts dry and slice them in half. Preheat the oven to 400°F.

2. In a small bowl, whisk together the maple syrup, olive oil, mustard, and salt to taste.

3. In a medium bowl, toss the sprouts with the maple mixture.

4. Spread the sprouts out in a single layer on a baking sheet. Roast for 20 minutes.

Makes 4 servings

Per serving: 146 calories, 4 g protein, 19 g carbohydrates, 7 g total fat (1 g saturated fat), 5 g fiber, 322 mg sodium

Beet Hummus

1   can (15.5 ounces) chickpeas, rinsed and drained
2   medium cooked beets, chopped
2   tablespoons fresh lemon juice
1½ tablespoons tahini
1½ tablespoons extra virgin olive oil
1   teaspoon chopped garlic
    Salt and ground black pepper
    Sweet potato chips

1. In a food processor, combine the chickpeas, beets, lemon juice, tahini, oil, and garlic. Puree until smooth. Season to taste with salt and pepper.

2. Serve the hummus with sweet potato chips.

Makes 4 servings

Per serving: 194 calories, 6 g protein, 24 g carbohydrates, 9 g total fat (1 g saturated fat), 5 g fiber, 124 mg sodium

Baked Beet Chips

3   medium beets, peeled and thinly sliced

1½ tablespoons coconut oil, melted

¼   teaspoon salt

1. Preheat the oven to 350°F.

2. In a bowl, toss the beets with the coconut oil and salt.

3. Spread the beets in a single layer on 2 baking sheets. Bake for 15 minutes. Flip the beets and bake for an additional 10 to 15 minutes, or until the beets have dried out and become crisp.

4. Cool before serving. The beet chips can be stored in an airtight container for up to 3 days.

Makes 6 servings

Per serving: 47 calories, 1 g protein, 4 g carbohydrates, 4 g total fat (3 g saturated fat), 1 g fiber, 129 mg sodium

Cantaloupe and Kiwi Pops

1   cup cantaloupe puree
1   cup kiwifruit puree (with seeds)
²⁄₃   cup simple syrup, divided
4   teaspoons lemon juice, divided
¼   cup Campari

1. Place the cantaloupe puree and kiwi puree into 2 separate bowls. Add ¹⁄₃ cup of the simple syrup and 2 teaspoons of the lemon juice to each bowl of fruit puree. Add the Campari to the cantaloupe mixture.

2. Pour the kiwi mixture into 8 juice bar molds, leaving room at the top.

3. Add sticks and freeze until firm, about 1 hour.

4. Pour the cantaloupe mixture on top of the kiwi layer and freeze. When firm, after at least 1 more hour, briefly dip the molds in warm water to loosen the pops before serving.

Makes 8 servings

Per serving: 50 calories, 0.5 g protein, 12 g carbohydrates, 0 g total fat (0 g saturated fat), 1 g fiber, 5 mg sodium

Date Energy Bites

7	pitted Medjool dates
¾	cup unsalted cashews
1	tablespoon flaxseeds
½	teaspoon almond extract
1	tablespoon water
¼	cup dried cranberries

1. In a food processor, combine the dates, cashews, flaxseeds, and almond extract. Process for 1 minute.

2. Add the water and dried cranberries and process until the mixture forms a ball.

3. Line a baking sheet with parchment paper. Scoop rounded table-spoons of the mixture onto the baking sheet and freeze. Once frozen, transfer the bites to a sealed container in the freezer until ready to serve.

4. Defrost before eating.

Makes 7 servings

Per serving: 171 calories, 3 g protein, 27 g carbohydrates, 7 g total fat (1 g saturated fat), 3 g fiber, 3 mg sodium

The Energy Booster

Potassium-rich bananas deliver energizing carbs, while protein powder and peanut butter give you energy to get through the three o'clock slump. Pantothenic acid, a B vitamin found in yogurt and honey, helps convert food into fuel. Iron-rich wheat germ and cinnamon pump up blood oxygen levels so you won't get winded during your midday workout.

2	frozen bananas, peeled and chopped
2	scoops chocolate protein powder
2	tablespoons peanut butter
2	tablespoons wheat germ
1	teaspoon ground cinnamon
1	tablespoon honey
¾	cup low-fat plain Greek yogurt
1	tablespoon skim milk powder
2	cups ice

In a blender, combine the bananas, protein powder, peanut butter, wheat germ, cinnamon, honey, yogurt, skim milk powder, and ice. Blend until smooth.

Makes 3 servings

Per serving: 294 calories, 25 g protein, 38 g carbohydrates, 7 g total fat (2 g saturated fat), 4 g fiber, 102 mg sodium

Cukes and Lime Jell-O

1   package (3 ounces) lime-flavored Jell-O
1   cup boiling water
1   cup low-fat, no-salt-added cottage cheese
1   cup fat-free plain yogurt
1   large cucumber, peeled, seeded, and coarsely grated (Option: If you use an English cucumber, you won't have to remove the seeds.)

1. In a large bowl,* combine the Jell-O and boiling water and stir until the gelatin is dissolved. Allow to sit for 5 minutes.

2. Refrigerate for 10 to 15 minutes, or until the gelatin begins to set.

3. Add the cottage cheese, yogurt, and cucumber. Whisk until well mixed and slightly frothy.

4. Refrigerate for 4 hours or overnight, until firm.

   * Or use a gelatin mold. First, lightly coat the mold with cooking spray, and then wipe off the excess oil with a paper towel before adding the Jell-O mixture. When the gelatin is fully set, invert it onto a serving plate.

Makes 6 servings

Per serving: 99 calories, 8 g protein, 17 g carbohydrates, 1/2 g total fat (0 g saturated fat), 0 g fiber, 93 mg sodium

How to Get More Protein in Your Diet

Protein is an essential macronutrient for building strength and muscle, but if you're not a big-time carnivore, you might be challenged to get enough into your diet, especially when it comes to your in-between meals, your snacks.

Protein supplements are a great option, except that the choices seem endless—there are plant-based protein powders, whey, hemp, casein, protein bars, gels, gummies—ah! How does one pick what's best? Review these general rules and you'll save yourself from experiencing chalky aftertastes, expending extra cash, and downing extra calories.

Decode Label Lingo

When shopping for supplements, avoid anything that claims to be a "meal replacement." While you know protein is an essential ingredient in every meal, it's only one piece of a well-rounded plate. One ingredient can't do all the work, and it certainly won't fill you up completely. I prefer to make protein shakes myself instead of relying on premade meal replacement shakes since they allow me to add more nutritious ingredients to my fuel. If you buy packaged food, do your best to avoid labels that mention artificial sweeteners, colors, or flavors within the first few ingredients.

Build Your Base

Protein powders are brilliant around workouts because they deliver fast-digesting protein to your muscles when they need it most. I lean on whey protein isolate and casein—both milk-based powders that pack in up to 25 grams of protein per scoop. Another great option is egg-white protein powder. It's the closest thing to "real food," made with natural ingredients and pure egg whites. If you don't do dairy, plant-based proteins such as pea protein (24 grams per scoop) and hemp protein (11 grams per scoop) are awesome alternatives. The rule of thumb on powders is to ensure they contain more grams of protein than any other nutrient.

Add an Enhancer

Combining protein with a fast-digesting carbohydrate speeds the delivery of protein to your muscles postworkout. Try adding a tablespoon of agave nectar to a scoop of vanilla whey protein powder and 8 ounces of water; you'll tally up 25 grams of protein in just 180 calories. If you have more time, try blending a banana with one scoop of chocolate whey protein powder and a tablespoon of all-natural nut butter (about 290 calories, 30 grams of protein).

Start with These Shake Recipes

Fruity Mega Mix

8	ounces water
½	teaspoon Crystal Light drink mix (try the "pure" tropical blend for flavor without artificial sweeteners)
10	ounces 1% milk
½	banana
	Handful of blueberries
	About 1 teaspoon pineapple juice, or a few pineapple chunks
2	scoops vanilla whey protein powder

Pour the water into a blender, followed by the drink mix and milk. Add the banana, blueberries, and pineapple juice or chunks. Finally, add vanilla protein powder (to complement the fruit), and mix until frothy.

Nutrition facts: 382 calories , 51 g protein, 41 g carbohydrates, 33 g sugar, 5 g fat

Supercharged Chocolate Shake

2	frozen bananas (peeled and chopped)
2	scoops chocolate protein powder
1	tablespoon peanut butter
2	tablespoons wheat germ
1	teaspoon ground cinnamon
¾	cup Greek yogurt
4	tablespoons skim milk powder
2	cups ice

Combine ingredients and blend until smooth.

Nutrition facts: 294 calories, 25 g protein, 38 g carbohydrates, 21 g sugar, 7 g fat

Java Jolt

¾	cup part-skim ricotta cheese
2	tablespoons Greek yogurt
1	tablespoon slivered, unsalted almonds
2	teaspoons chocolate whey protein powder
2	teaspoons ground flaxseeds
½	teaspoon finely ground coffee beans
6	ice cubes

Chuck everything into a blender. Mix well.

Nutrition facts: 185 calories, 15 g protein, 10 g carbohydrates, 3 g sugar, 10 g fat

Breakfast Blend

¾	cup instant oatmeal, nuked in water or fat-free milk
¾	cup fat-free milk
¾	cup mixed berries (blue are best for a jolt of antioxidants)
2	teaspoons vanilla whey protein powder
3	ice cubes, crushed

Include all ingredients in a blender, and blend until smooth. For a thicker texture, add more ice.

Nutrition facts: 122 calories, 9 g protein, 20 g carbohydrates, 9 g sugar, 1.5 g fat

(continued)

For more ideas, check out the recipes at womenshealthmag.com/nutrition.

Pass the Bar

Too busy to blend? I keep a protein bar on hand for days I can't seem to slow down. Regardless of the brand, always check the back before buying. Protein bars easily go awry with added sugar, artificial sweeteners, sugar alcohol, and protein substitutes like gelatin and hydrolyzed collagen. Keep things simple: Aim for a bar with 100 to 200 calories, with at least 6 grams of protein (*at the top of the ingredient list*), fewer than 35 grams of carbs (*no more than 19 from sugar*), about 5 grams of fiber, and with calcium.

Get Real

If you're on the road and only have time to make pit stops, make sure you choose the best option available. Shakes and bars are great if you're stuck in the driver's seat, but if you're riding shotgun, go for Greek yogurt, beef jerky, or a hard-cooked egg. You won't have to spend 15 minutes deciphering dense labels, and most convenience stores stock them.

To round out your arsenal of protein-rich shakes, bars, and convenience-food store snacks, try these quick and easy mini meals made at home.

Baby carrots and hummus

Carrots contain complex carbs to sustain your energy levels, and provide enough potassium to control blood pressure and muscle contractions. Add 2 tablespoons of hummus to your mini meal for slow-digesting carbs, protein, and unsaturated fats—all the right elements to fuel activity. Plus, most varieties are made with olive oil, which contains oleic acid—a fat that aids in warding off the gene responsible for 20 to 30 percent of breast cancers, according to research from Northwestern University.

Half cup of edamame and a stick of reduced-fat string cheese

Sargento String Cheese Snacks keep your calories in check with 8 grams of protein in just 80 calories. Add edamame for another 9 grams of protein and a dose of heart-healthy omega-3 fatty acids.

PB&J

Remix your lunch box fave. Spread a tablespoon of natural peanut butter on sprouted grain Ezekiel bread. Top with a handful of sliced strawberries instead of jelly for a mini meal that contains 10 grams of protein in less than 200 calories.

PB&Cheese

Not sure if you want something sweet, salty, or cheesy? Surprisingly, you can have all three—and be healthy! Try 2 tablespoons of natural peanut butter on a whole grain English muffin with 1 stick of part-skim string cheese (torn into strands). The result is a mess-free mini meal with 23 grams of protein.

Two leaves of lettuce with light cheese and sliced turkey

Roll a Laughing Cow light cheese and 2 thin slices of deli turkey into a large lettuce leaf. Pack two for a low-fat meal that tallies up 25 grams of protein in 160 calories.

Cottage cheese with pumpkin seeds and cereal

Be sure to pack a spoon. Two tablespoons of pumpkin seeds and $\frac{1}{2}$ cup Kashi Go Lean cereal on top of $\frac{1}{2}$ cup cottage cheese satisfies your need for crunch and savory flavor. The seeds supply omega-3s, magnesium, and iron to fuel your muscle recovery. The combo with Kashi and cottage cheese pumps your protein intake up to 25 grams in one dish.

Lift to Get Lean

Acknowledgments

This book is the culmination of trials and errors, discoveries, and especially relationships. It's been an incredible journey, and I'm honored to wake up every day and inspire people to live a better life through fitness. I thank you, cherish you, and celebrate every one of you.

Trampas Thompson, there isn't enough space here to express my appreciation for your support, cheerleading, and unconditional love, all of which helped me find my voice. You were the one who encouraged me to write my first magazine article, and look where we've arrived.

Thank you...

> To Amy Stanton, for paving the road to this book. You're a thoughtful leader, creative mind, and masterful networker.

> To Michele Promaulayko, for asking me to contribute to your book *20 Pounds Younger,* which ultimately led to this book opportunity. You're a champion for women, an inspiration, and a trendsetter. And your support for strength training for women helped to cause a shift in thinking that will benefit women for years to come.

> To *Women's Health* magazine. Your writers and editors rise above the rest to check facts and report honest, accurate information that women can use to improve their lives in so many ways. Thank you for letting me be a part of a talented team of journalists.

> To the editors and designers at Rodale Books, including Jeff Csatari, executive editor of *Women's Health* books; Amy Rushlow; Hope Clarke; Joanna Williams; Gillian Francella; and photographer Tom MacDonald. I am a trainer by day, so it helped immensely to have a team of professionals guide, inspire, and massage my message and instruction to make it easier to follow and more useful.

> To Jill Esplin, Lani Slagle Wille, Kelli Perkins, Cindy de La Cruz, and Trampas, thank you for being my tribe—your love and support help me better serve my clients and readers.

> To Mom and Dad. Thank you for every little thing I may have forgotten to thank you for over the years, especially for encouraging me to go to college. You knew I was needed for something bigger in this world. I love you.

> To all my clients since 1996. Thank you for allowing me to guide your health, learn from you, and develop the philosophies that shaped my career and this book.

> To Pat Manocchia, who showed me that fitness is about much more than being fit. You taught me that putting one foot in front of the other creates the momentum and strength to climb mountains.

> To Karl Stoedefalke, a true pioneer of the fitness industry. My life changed the moment I first sat in your class at Penn State. The passion (and legitimacy) you brought to being a fitness professional inspired my own love for this vocation.

> Finally, I feel exceptionally honored to be a part of New Balance, a company with impeccable standards and passionate team members. Thank you for every experience we've shared over the past 7 years and for filling my closet with sneakers to support all my running, jumping, and squatting every day!

Appendix

Workout Log

DATE: _____   TODAY'S WEIGHT: _____

EXERCISE	SETS	REPS	TIME	WEIGHT	NOTES

Photocopy these pages so you can log your results at the gym.

Workout Log

DATE: _____ TODAY'S WEIGHT: _____

EXERCISE	SETS	REPS	TIME	WEIGHT	NOTES

DATE: _____ TODAY'S WEIGHT: _____

EXERCISE	SETS	REPS	TIME	WEIGHT	NOTES

Workout Log

DATE: TODAY'S WEIGHT:

EXERCISE	SETS	REPS	TIME	WEIGHT	NOTES

DATE: TODAY'S WEIGHT:

EXERCISE	SETS	REPS	TIME	WEIGHT	NOTES

Workout Log

DATE: _____   TODAY'S WEIGHT: _____

EXERCISE	SETS	REPS	TIME	WEIGHT	NOTES

DATE: _____   TODAY'S WEIGHT: _____

EXERCISE	SETS	REPS	TIME	WEIGHT	NOTES

Workout Log

DATE: TODAY'S WEIGHT:

EXERCISE	SETS	REPS	TIME	WEIGHT	NOTES

DATE: TODAY'S WEIGHT:

EXERCISE	SETS	REPS	TIME	WEIGHT	NOTES

Workout Log

DATE: _____ TODAY'S WEIGHT: _____

EXERCISE	SETS	REPS	TIME	WEIGHT	NOTES

DATE: _____ TODAY'S WEIGHT: _____

EXERCISE	SETS	REPS	TIME	WEIGHT	NOTES

Workout Log

DATE: _____ TODAY'S WEIGHT: _____

EXERCISE	SETS	REPS	TIME	WEIGHT	NOTES

DATE: _____ TODAY'S WEIGHT: _____

EXERCISE	SETS	REPS	TIME	WEIGHT	NOTES

Workout Log

DATE: _____ TODAY'S WEIGHT: _____

EXERCISE	SETS	REPS	TIME	WEIGHT	NOTES

DATE: _____ TODAY'S WEIGHT: _____

EXERCISE	SETS	REPS	TIME	WEIGHT	NOTES

Index

Boldface page references indicate photographs. Underscored references indicate boxed text.